Gary McCleane, MD

Cholecystokinin and Its Antagonists in Pain Management

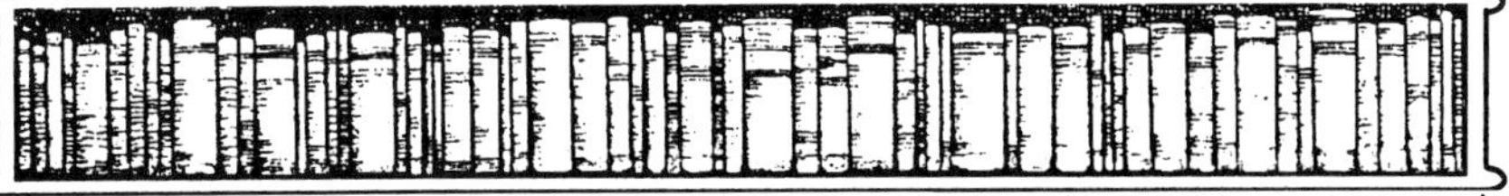

Cholecystokinin
and Its Antagonists
in Pain Management

The Haworth Medical Press®
Haworth Series in Clinical Pain and Symptom Palliation
Senior Editor Howard Smith

Clinical Management of the Elderly Patient in Pain
edited by Gary McCleane and Howard Smith

Cholecystokinin and Its Antagonists in Pain Management
by Gary McCleane

Titles of Related Interest

*Pain and Palliative Care in the Developing World and Marginalized
Populations: A Global Challenge* edited by M.R. Rojogopal,
David Mazza, and Arthur J. Lipman

Aging, Spirituality, and Palliative Care by Elizabeth MacKinlay

Chronic Pain: Biomedical and Spiritual Approaches by Harold G. Koenig

Concise Encyclopedia of Pain Psychology by Roger B. Fillingim

*Autogenic Training: A Mind-Body Approach to the Treatment
of Fibromyalgia and Chronic Pain Syndrome* by Micah R. Sadigh

The Concise Encyclopedia of Fibromyalgia and Myofascial Pain
by Roberto Patarca-Montero

Cholecystokinin and Its Antagonists in Pain Management

Gary McCleane, MD

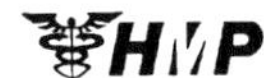

The Haworth Medical Press®
An Imprint of The Haworth Press, Inc.
New York • London • Oxford

Library of Congress Cataloging-in-Publication Data

McCleane, Gary.
   Cholecystokinin and its antagonists in pain management / Gary McCleane.
      p. ; cm.
   Includes bibliographical references and index.
   ISBN-13: 978-0-7890-2892-1 (hard : alk. paper)
   ISBN-10: 0-7890-2892-1 (hard : alk. paper)
   ISBN-13: 978-0-7890-2893-8 (soft : alk. paper)
   ISBN-10: 0-7890-2893-X (soft : alk. paper)
      1. Cholecystokinin—Antagonists—Therapeutic use. 2. Cholecystokinin—Physiological effect. 3. Pain—Chemotherapy. [DNLM: 1. Cholecystokinin—antagonists & inhibitors. 2. Cholecysto-kinin—secretion. 3. Cholecystokinin—therapeutic use. 4. Analgesics, Opioid—pharmacokinetics. 5. Analgesics, Opioid—therapeutic use. 6. Pain—drug therapy. WK 170 M478c 2006] I. Title.

QP572.C5.M33 2006
616'.0472—dc22

                                                                              2005037761

CONTENTS

ABOUT THE AUTHOR

Gary McCleane, MD, is a United Kingdom-based consultant in pain management. He has published widely in the field of treatment options for neuropathic pain. Among his research interests are the clinical application of cholecystokinin antagonists in human pain management. He has conducted a number of studies with cholecystokinin antagonists and confirmed a useful role for this class of agent in pain management.

Chapter 1

Introduction

Much has changed in our understanding of the pathophysiology and treatment of pain in the past few years. To a certain extent this increase in knowledge has led to the introduction of new therapeutic agents and improved our ability to provide pain relief. Yet there are still many patients, particularly with chronic pain conditions, who we fail to provide with adequate pain relief or on whom we impose unpleasant side effects with the analgesic treatment.

Given what we now know about many receptors, ion channels, pathways, and neural structures that are intimately involved in pain processing, it should be of no surprise that malfunction can occur at any of these areas following tissue injury. This may lead to chronic pain. Any one therapeutic agent with a distinct and defined mode of action may not be efficacious in lessening the pain maintained by such malfunctioning in every sufferer. The need to have a range of therapeutic options, each with a distinct and different mode of action so as to cover ever eventuality, is clear. That said, if there are ways in which we can either increase the quality of analgesia produced by a drug, or achieve the same level of analgesia with a smaller dose, thereby reducing side effects, this would be advantageous. Furthermore, if there are strategies we can institute to ensure that the initial level of analgesia provided by an agent is maintained without the need to increase dose with the passage of time, this too would be advantageous. Significant evidence from animal experimentation suggests that the cholecystokinin antagonists may possess some of these desirable characteristics when used in conjunction with opioid analgesics. They seem to be able to enhance the quality of opioid-derived antinociception when used in animals with the added properties of seeming to attenuate antinociceptive

Cholecystokinin and Its Antagonists in Pain Management
© 2006 by The Haworth Press, Inc. All rights reserved.
doi:10.1300/5593_01

tolerance and even to reverse established tolerance. The human work that has been done, although sparse, seems to support, to a certain extent, these animal findings and confirm that the addition of a cholecystokinin antagonist to an opioid is an intervention with a low risk.

Perhaps now more than ever, we should be focusing on therapeutic options that can increase the efficacy and long-term safety of opioid analgesics given the increased availability of a variety of strong opioid analgesics in clinical practice and the apparent decrease in the threshold for their use. No longer are strong opioids used only in the treatment of acute pain or that associated with terminal illnesses. Now it is not unusual for such strong opioids to be used as a treatment for the pain produced by chronic disease processes such as osteo-arthritis, low back pain, and postherpetic neuralgia.

Therefore, it is proposed, that cholecystokinin antagonists may have a role in enhancing the quality of analgesia produced by opioid analgesics and in reducing the analgesic tolerance that can occur when opioids are used in the long term. The forthcoming chapters will show compelling evidence that supports this proposition. This will be supported by a review of the role of opioids in pain management and an insight into the functioning of cholecystokinin in both health and disease. Why this evidence has not been translated into the clinical availability of cholecystokinin antagonists has many reasons. Among these is the fact that cholecystokinin antagonists, by and large, were synthesised many years ago and any patent protection that could be obtained has since expired. Therefore, the pharmaceutical industry seems unwilling to invest in the verification of these agents in clinical practice, a necessary step prior to licensing when the concept and drug under investigation have no patent protection. Clinical experience suggests that available cholecystokinin antagonists have a degree of efficacy and safety profile superior to many other recently licensed preparations. This knowledge set against the backdrop of restricted clinical availability is frustrating.

If assessment of the available literature surrounding the effects of cholecystokinin and its antagonists in pain management supports the contention that cholecystokinin antagonists have a useful role in pain management then it could be envisaged that opioids, whether weak or strong, could be presented as combination products containing a cholecystokinin antagonist. After all, why use an opioid alone when the addition of a cholecystokinin antagonist has the potential for both enhancing the analgesia produced by the opioid and minimizing the risk of analgesic tolerance and yet not adding to the side effects that may be apparent with use of the opioid alone?

Chapter 2

Opioids in Pain Management

Perhaps the most extensively used class of drugs in pain management is the opioids. These drugs bind to specific opioid receptors found both centrally and peripherally. In cases where the receptor affinity is low, the drug in question is known as a "weak" opioid; where the receptor affinity is stronger, the opioid is known as a "strong" opioid. Although the use of weak opioids in the form of, for example, codeine is extensive, it is only more recently that more extensive use has been made of the stronger members of this class. One of the most significant steps forward in the management of pain associated with terminal illness has been a realization of the value of strong opioids, as indicated in the World Health Organization "ladder approach" to management. This progress has been strengthened by the increasing availability of extended-release strong opioids in either oral or transdermal preparations.

In other pain conditions, the acceptance of the use of strong opioids has been slower. Only now is it clear that strong opioids can have an effect in, for example, neuropathic pain.[1,2]

The pharmacological effects of the opioid analgesics are derived from the complex interactions with three opioid receptor types (mu, delta, and kappa). These receptors are found in the periphery, at presynaptic and postsynaptic sites in the spinal cord dorsal horn, and in the brainstem, thalamus, and cortex in what constitutes the ascending pain transmission system, as well as structures that comprise a descending inhibitory system which modulates pain at the level of the spinal cord. The cellular effects of opioids include a decrease in presynaptic transmitter release, hyperpolarization of postsynaptic elements, and disinhibition.[3-5] At high concentrations opioids can inhibit N-methy-D-aspartate receptor channels[6] and decrease excitatory neurotransmitter release from primary nociceptive neurons, an

Cholecystokinin and Its Antagonists in Pain Management
© 2006 by The Haworth Press, Inc. All rights reserved.
doi:10.1300/5593_02

effect that may be due to inhibition of presynaptic voltage-activated calcium channels.[7]

CODEINE

Despite extensive clinical use, the evidence validating the analgesic effect of codeine is sparse. In one of the few randomized, controlled trials, Peloso and colleagues (2000) examined the effect of codeine in patients with osteoarthritis of the hips and knees. They found codeine to be significantly more efficacious in terms of its analgesic effect and effect on stiffness than placebo.[8] In a study of the effect of codeine in human experimental pain, Enggaard and colleagues (2001) were able to show that codeine inhibited temporal summation (pain summation at tolerance threshold to repetitive electrical sural nerve stimulation), a feature of neuropathic pain.[9] Moore and colleagues (1997) calculated (from the studies available at that time) that the "numbers needed to treat" (NNT) for codeine 60 mg when used for postoperative pain as 9.1.[10]

Codeine itself has little or no analgesic effect. It requires O-demethylation to morphine to achieve its full analgesic potential. This conversion is mediated by cytochrome P450 2D6 in humans.[11] A proportion of the population lacks this enzyme[12] and hence derive no analgesia from codeine. Similarly, these patients can be expected not to get withdrawal reactions when codeine treatment is terminated.[13]

DIHYDROCODEINE

Unlike codeine, dihydrocodeine has intrinsic analgesic properties and CYP2D6 phenotype has no impact on dihydrocodeine-derived analgesia.[14,15] Dihydrocodeine is metabolized to dihydromorphine, dihydrocodeine-6-O and dihydromorphine-3-O- and dihydromorphine-6-O-glucuronide and nordihydrocodeine. These metabolites have a high affinity for mu opioid receptors and have analgesic effects.[16]

TRAMADOL

Tramadol shares both effects on central mu opioid receptors and inhibition of noradrenaline and serotonin reuptake.[17] Tramadol has been shown to be effective in relieving pain from a variety of sources including osteoarthritis pain,[18,19] diabetic neuropathy,[20] postherpetic neuralgia,[21] and painful polyneuropathy.[22] Its effect on neuropathic pain may be due to its combined opioid and monoaminergic effects.[23] Adler and colleagues (2002) have shown that when used for the treatment of osteoarthritis pain, similar levels of analgesia are achieved with both normal release and extended-release tramadol preparations, but that the extended-relief preparations produce this relief at a lower dose.[24]

MORPHINE

Despite over two centuries of use as an analgesic, it is only in recent times that morphine has been used as an analgesic in nonacute situations. In the case of neuropathic pain, this reluctance to consider long-term use of morphine, and other strong opioids, was most acute. Now it is becoming clear that morphine can reduce neuropathic pain[25-27] as well as the pain associated with other chronic conditions such as osteoarthritis.[28] In many chronic pain states, use of morphine is associated not only with a reduction in pain, but also with improvement in physical function, depression, mood, and exercise tolerance.[29] The advent of sustained-release oral preparations,[30] rectal,[31,32] and even nasal morphine,[33] has increased the range of situations in which morphine has advantages.

OXYCODONE

As with morphine, evidence suggests that oxycodone can relieve, for example, osteoarthritis pain[34] as well as that associated with diabetic neuropathy and postherpetic neuralgia.[35,36] Oxycodone is not a new drug, although its presentation as an extended-release preparation is a recent innovation. Some argue that its clinical effect is not much different than that of morphine.[37]

FENTANYL

Fentanyl, an opioid with a relatively short half-life when given parenterally or orally in an immediate-release formulation, has been extensively used in anaesthetic practice where it has gained popularity because of its predictable duration of action and efficacy. Only in recent times has its use extended to other fields. Dellemijn and Vanneste (1997) compared the analgesic effect of intravenous fentanyl with intravenous diazepam (an active comparator) and placebo in patients with neuropathic pain of various etiologies. They demonstrated a useful analgesic effect when fentanyl was given by the intravenous route.[38] Given that intravenous fentanyl has a rapid analgesic effect, and hence can be titrated to effect, it can be used for the rapid management of cancer-related pain.[39] Bredenberg and colleagues (2003) have described the use of a sublingual formulation of fentanyl and shown that it is rapidly absorbed and could therefore be expected to have a rapid onset of action.[40] Indeed, even nebulized fentanyl can be used in the management of acute pain.[41]

Although this quick onset of effect has definite advantages in certain defined circumstances, this quick effect can be matched by a rapid cessation of effect, a property with definite disadvantages when managing all but the most acute of pains. The formulation of an extended-release transdermal fentanyl patch has had a major impact in dealing with pain of longer duration. This patch delivers a defined amount of fentanyl (25, 50, or 75 µg/hour) over 72 hours. Because of its short half-life, the time to steady state is relatively short. Transdermal fentanyl has been shown to be effective in cancer-related pain,[42-44] chronic pain,[45] postoperative pain,[46] and the pain associated with vertebral collapse fractures,[47] among others.

In comparison to other strong opioids, van Seventer and colleagues (2003) found that in patients with moderate-to-severe cancer-related pain, transdermal fentanyl was as efficacious as extended-release morphine but with fewer side effects.[48]

Though the rate of dermal penetration of fentanyl is variable in humans, penetration from the transdermal patches currently in use is associated with less variability.[49]

HYDROMORPHONE

Quigley (2002) has assessed the available studies relating to the use of hydromorphone in acute and chronic pain. Forty-three studies were considered: half were found to be of low quality. Only three were placebo controlled. In the others, hydromorphone was compared with other strong opioids. He concluded that "the majority demonstrated that hydromorphone is a potent analgesic, that the clinical effects of hydromorphone appear to be dose-related, and that the adverse effect profile of hydromorphone is similar to that of other mu opioid receptor agonists."[50]

BUPRENORPHINE

Buprenorphine is a low-molecular-weight, lipophilic, opioid analgesic with a kappa opioid receptor effect. Previously available as a sublingual and parenteral formulation, buprenorphine is now presented as a transdermal patch delivering 35, 52.5, or 70 µg/hour over a 72-hour period. Initial reports confirm an analgesic effect that would be expected from such an opioid with increased patient satisfaction over the previously available forms of buprenorphine.[51-53]

Although it is beyond doubt that opioids are useful in the treatment of a whole range of pain conditions, they are neither universally efficacious nor well tolerated. One possible approach to inadequate pain relief or intolerable side effects is for conversion from one opioid to another on a sequential basis, so-called "opioid rotation." This is suggested by some as a useful maneuver,[54] although Quigley (2004), having analyzed the available studies has concluded that "the evidence to support the practice of switching is largely anecdotal or based on observational and uncontrolled studies."[55]

Although the efficacy of opioids, be they weak or strong, is important, their tolerability is also a major factor. Opioid-induced side effects may be immediately apparent, slower in onset, or be so insidious as to be apparent only on careful examination. Perhaps one of the most common side effects associated with opioid use is constipation. Staats and colleagues (2004) retrospectively studied 1,836 patients receiving treatment with transdermal fentanyl, sustained-release oxycodone, and sustained-release morphine. Those receiving transdermal fentanyl had a lower risk of developing constipation than those taking either of the other two strong opioids (3 percent as opposed to a 6 percent risk with oxycodone and 5 percent with morphine).[56] The incidence for the occurrence of constipation is significantly lower than others report with transdermal fentanyl. For example, Milligan and colleagues (2001) found that with transdermal fentanyl use over a

12-month period in an open-label trial in which 301 patients continued use for the 12 months, constipation was noted as a side effect in 19 percent.[57] Menten and colleagues (2002) suggest that in terms of patients treated with transdermal fentanyl for cancer-related pain, the incidence of constipation is related not to the dose of transdermal fentanyl used, but rather on the amount of morphine used as a rescue analgesic.[58] Van Seventer and colleagues (2003) give support to the impression of a lower risk of constipation with transdermal fentanyl. They enrolled 131 patients and commenced them on transdermal fentanyl or controlled-release morphine. Doses were titrated until effect was apparent. The quality of analgesia achieved in both groups was equal. Constipation was less common in those treated with fentanyl: at the end of one week, 27 percent in the fentanyl group reported constipation as opposed to 57 percent in the controlled-release morphine group. In general terms, other side effects were more common, or severe, in the morphine group. Of the patients enrolled in the study, 36 percent in the controlled-release morphine group withdrew because of side effects as opposed to only 4 percent in the transdermal fentanyl group. Of those who continued with the trial, 14 percent in the fentanyl group reported troublesome side effects as opposed to 36 percent in the morphine group.[59] Efficacy and incidence of side effects seems to be, at least in part, dose related.[60] Furthermore, the incidence of side effects decreases with sustained use.[61] With extended-release preparations, these side effects may be more gradual in onset, as may be their initial analgesic effect. That said, Watson and colleagues (2003) studied patients with painful diabetic neuropathy. Patients were treated for four weeks with controlled-release oxycodone or placebo. The only side effects that occurred on a statistically more significant basis in the oxycodone-treated group were dry mouth and constipation.[62]

A recurrent anxiety associated with chronic strong opioid administration is its effect on cognition and motor tasks as exemplified by driving safety. Schindler and colleagues (2004) examined this issue in opioid addicts (not with chronic pain) using an Austrian standard test battery for measurement of performance related to driving ability, the Act & React Test (ART) system. Subjects were taking either methadone or buprenorphine and were compared to healthy controls. They found that those taking these strong opioids did not differ significantly in comparison with the healthy controls in the majority of the ART standard tests.[63]

Jamison and colleagues (2003) examined the psychomotor effects of long-term opioid (oxycodone and fentanyl) use in 144 patients with low back pain. They measured the results of two neuropsychological tests (Digit Symbol and Trail Making Test-B) on all subjects prior to institution of the strong opioid and again 90 and 180 days after opioid commencement. They found that sustained use was not associated with impairment of the neuropsychological variables measured. Indeed, memory, incidental learning, and psychomotor performance were improved in many of the subjects. They also noted that a minority of patients had a decrease in performance. This tended to occur in older patients and in those with lower pretreatment pain scores. There were no differences in neuropsychological performance between patients taking oxycodone or transdermal fentanyl.[64]

Tassain and colleagues (2003) studied 28 patients with chronic noncancer pain in whom sustained-release morphine was prescribed. Eighteen stayed on this therapy and the other ten discontinued treatment because of unacceptable side effects but acted as a control group. They found that when baseline, pretreatment neuropsychological variables were compared in these patients with results obtained after 3, 6, and 12 months treatment that there were no significant differences. In two measures of information processing (the Stroop interference score and the digit symbol test) the results were actually better after 6 and 12 months treatment. The most frequent side effects with treatment were gastrointestinal in nature with almost 50 percent of patients still reporting constipation after 12 months of morphine therapy.[65]

Similarly, Sabatowski and colleagues (2003) measured attention, reaction, visual orientation, motor coordination, and vigilance in 30 subjects using a stable dose of transdermal fentanyl for noncancer pain and compared these to 90 healthy volunteers. None of the results from the measures differed significantly between the fentanyl-treated and volunteer subjects and they concluded that in patients treated with stable doses of transdermal fentanyl, the threshold for fitness to drive did not differ significantly between the groups.[66]

In contrast, when morphine and OxyContin were administered on a one-off basis to volunteers and compared to placebo, both morphine and oxycontin produced effects on psychomotor performance and these effects were dose related.[67]

Longer-term administration may be complicated by other factors that can influence their long-term tolerability. For example, acute administration of opioids increases prolactin, growth hormone, thyroid-stimulating hormone, and ACTH while inhibiting leutenizing hormone (LH) release.[68-70] When administered on a long-term basis, different endocrine results are observed. Abs and colleagues (2000) extensively investigated 73 patients receiving intrathecal opioids for chronic, nonmalignant pain. Average duration of opioid treatment was 26 months. Decreased libido and impotence was present in 23 of the 24 men studied. Nine of the men had a significantly reduced testosterone level and most had a decreased LH level. All of the premenopausal females had either amenorrhea or an irregular cycle with ovulation in only one patient. All postmenopausal women had a decreased LH and follicle-stimulating hormone (FSH) level when compared to controls. The twenty-four-hour urinary cortisol excretion was significantly lower than controls in 14 of the 73 patients. Fifteen percent of all patients developed growth hormone deficiency. Therefore, in patients receiving intrathecal opioids on a long-term basis, the majority of men and all women developed hypogonadotrophic hypogonadism, 15 percent developed central hypocorticism, and about 15 percent developed growth hormone deficiency.[71]

A single case report highlights a different possible side effect of fentanyl use. Kokko and colleagues (2002) reported apparent inappropriate antidiuretic hormone (ADH) release in a patient with a known lung tumor treated with fentanyl. Withdrawal of fentanyl terminated the ADH release, while reinstitution of fentanyl at a later date triggered of a further inappropriate ADH release.[72]

As with tricyclic antidepressants (TCAs), paradoxical pain can complicate opioid use.[73-85] If such pain occurs and remains unidentified, it may lead to an increase in opioid dose with a potential increase in opioid-related side effects and consequent reduction in tolerability. Opioid-induced paradoxical pain may be caused by opioid-induced release of spinal dynorphin and cholecystokinin.[86-90]

CONCLUSIONS

The evidence that opioids, both weak and strong, are effective in a wide variety of pain conditions is strong. However, they are not effective nor always the wisest choice in every patient. Even when they are effective, their use is at times complicated by a variety of side effects which precludes further use. The incidence and severity of side effects is often dose related. Maintenance of analgesic effect may necessitate a gradual dose increase as time progresses with consequent increase in these side effects. When opioids are titrated until a dose is reached in which analgesia is achieved and steady state is reached, some of the more concerning opioid-related side effects such as cognitive impairment cease to be problematical. Indeed, if pain relief is achieved in a patient with a chronic pain condition, this can be rewarded by an improvement in mood, functional ability, and overall quality of life. The safety of strong opioids, when used in all but the most acute of situations, has increased with the availability of extended-release preparations, be they with oral morphine or oxycodone or with the transdermal forms of fentanyl or buprenorphine.

Despite the increasing acceptance of the use of opioids in all pain conditions, problems still occur with their use. These include failure to produce useful analgesia in all patients, incomplete analgesia in others, and unacceptable side effects. To an extent, all of these may be dependent on the dose of opioid used. Increasing the dose may increase the proportion of patients getting relief and the extent of that relief. Conversely, dose escalation may increase the incidence and severity of side effects with a negative effect on the overall acceptability of opioid treatment.

Over time, many strategies have been suggested for improving the quantity of patients deriving analgesia and the quality of that analgesia from opioid use. The focus of this book is on the relationship between cholecystokinin and opioid-derived analgesia and how the use of cholecystokinin antagonists may represent a low-risk strategy for maximizing the efficaciousness of opioids.

Chapter 3

Cholecystokinin

THE ORIGINAL DESCRIPTION OF CHOLECYSTOKININ

The original use of the term "cholecystokinin" comes from the work of Ivy and Oldberg (1928). They used it to describe a hormonal substance that "excites or moves the gallbladder."[1]

Influenced by the work of Boyden (1926)[2] who found that transfusion of blood from fed cats into other cats caused partial evacuation of the gallbladder, they devised a series of experiments to elucidate the cause of this gallbladder contraction. For these experiments they used, among other things, a "purified" extract of the intestinal mucosa which was known as "secretin."

In the first of their experiments, they anesthetized cats, and cannulated the common bile duct and gallbladder. The gallbladder cannula was joined to a manometer from which pressure readings were taken. On intravenous injection of secretin the gallbladder pressure increased. After several minutes the flow of bile also increased. At no time was there any alteration in blood pressure or respiratory rate in the experimental animals. When saline was administered intravenously, no increase in gallbladder pressure or flow of bile was observed. To determine if the increase in gallbladder pressure was caused by the increased flow of bile, they performed similar experiments on cats whose cystic ducts had been clamped. Gallbladder pressure did increase in these animals, but not to the extent observed in unclamped animals.

Ivy and Oldberg proceeded to repeat this experiment in dogs. This time the gallbladder was cannulated (to allow pressure measurement) along with the pancreatic duct. With a single intravenous injection of secretin, gallbladder pressure increased after one to two minutes in all

Cholecystokinin and Its Antagonists in Pain Management

doi:10.1300/5593_03

15

but one of 80 dogs used in their experiments. This increase in gallbladder pressure occurred before pancreatic secretion had begun. They found that the duration of gallbladder contraction ranged from 10 to 60 minutes with an average of around 15 minutes. If the animals had been fed immediately prior to anesthesia, cannulation and secretin administration, then gallbladder contraction, were significantly less.

Ivy and Oldberg then proceeded to insert cannulae into the gallbladders of anesthetized dogs. In addition, their cystic ducts were clamped. Hydrochloric acid was injected into the duodenum. In every case studied, gallbladder contraction followed hydrochloric acid instillation. When olive oil, cream, or egg yolk was placed in the duodenum, no gallbladder contraction occurred. However, if the cream, olive oil, or egg yolk were digested with "pancreatin" prior to insertion in the duodenum, then gallbladder contraction did occur.

To gain further insight into the mechanisms involved, Ivy and Oldberg performed cross-circulation experiments. They connected the medial carotids in pairs of anesthetized dogs. Their cystic ducts were clamped, and their gallbladders and pancreatic ducts cannulated. In three of their four experiments, instillation of hydrochloric acid into the duodenum of the first dog caused the gallbladder to contract in the second animal. This contraction did not last as long in the second dog as the first. They felt this was due to a "dilution" of that substance released by the first dog in the blood of the second.

Ivy and Oldberg concluded that a substance released after stimulation by secretin or hydrochloric acid was causing the gallbladder to contract and express its contents. That this was not choline was proven by the failure of atropine to block the response; that it was not histamine by the lack of change in blood pressure. They named this substance "cholecystokinin" and felt that the results of their cross-circulation experiments suggested that it was a hormonal substance.

Following the work of Ivy and Oldberg (1928), Harper and Raper (1943) demonstrated that similar intestinal extracts contained a hormonal factor that, on intravenous administration, stimulated pancreatic enzyme secretion and proposed the name pancreozymin (PZ).[3]

In 1971, Mutt and Jorpes isolated a 33 amino acid polypeptide that had the properties of both cholecystokinin (CCK) and PZ and thus revealed that the two distinct hormones were, in fact, a single hormone.[4,5] Since CCK activity was the first described, the acronym CCK is now used instead of PZ or CCK-PZ.

MOLECULAR CHARACTERISTICS OF CHOLECYSTOKININ

Species-specific molecular variants of the amino acid sequence of CCK have been identified (see Figure 3.1). The 33 amino acid sequence and its eight amino C-terminal have been demonstrated in pigs, rats, chickens, chinchillas, dogs, and humans.[6-8] A 39 amino acid sequence has been found in pigs,[9] dogs,[10] and guinea pigs.[11] A 58 amino acid sequence has been reported in cats, dogs, and humans.[12] Frogs and turtles show 47 amino acid sequences homologous to CCK and to gastrin.[13] The nonsulphated octapeptide has been reported in rat brain.[14] The C-terminal pentapeptide conserves the

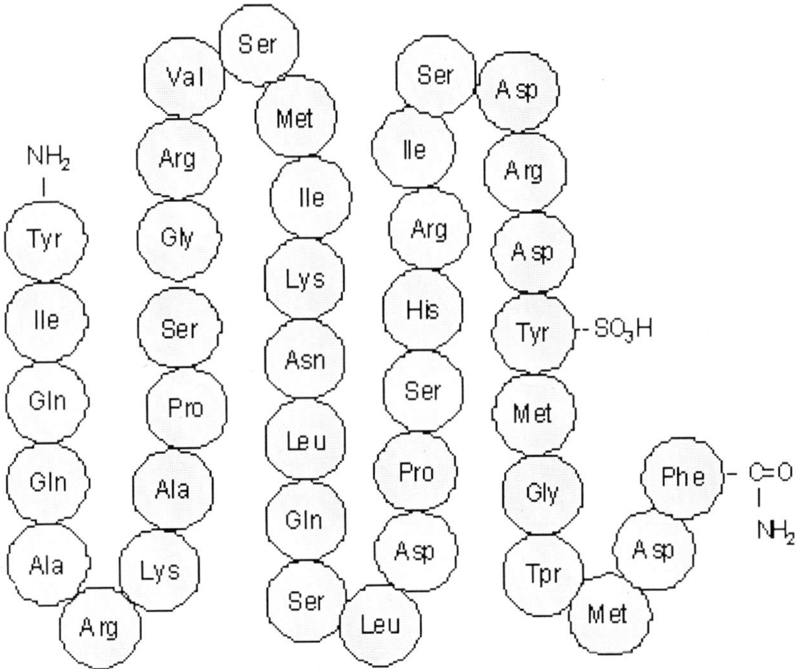

FIGURE 3.1. The amino acid sequence of porcine cholecystokinin. (*Sources:* Mutt V, Jorpes JE. Structure of porcine cholecystokinin-pancreozymin. Cleavage with thrombin and with trypsin. *Eur J Biochem* 1968; 6: 156-162; Deschenes RJ, Lorenz LJ, Haun RS, Roos BA, Collier KJ, Dixon JE. Cloning and sequence analysis of a cDNA encoding rat preprocholecystokinin in pig brain and gut. *Proc Natl Acad Sci USA* 1984; 81: 4307-4310.)

structural homology of the CCK sequences and also the homology of the neuropeptide gastrin.[7] The C-terminal sulphated octapeptide sequence Asp-Tyr(SO_3H)-Met-Gly-Trp-Met-Asp-Phe-NH_2 is relatively conserved across species and appears to be the minimal sequence for biological activity in rodents.[9,15]

In the next chapters we will see that CCK binds at two distinct receptors. This binding is saturable and reversible. These receptors can be differentiated by their affinity for the sulphated and nonsulphated eight terminal sequence of CCK. Sulphated CCK-8 has a much higher affinity for peripheral, alimentary tract CCK receptors than the unsulphated variety.[16-18] Sulphated CCK-8 is approximately 1,000 times more potent than unsulphated CCK-8 in stimulating pancreatic secretion.[17,19] In homogenates of cerebral cortex, CCK receptor binding is displaced by unsulphated CCK-8 at concentrations tenfold greater than sulphated CCK-8.[16,17,19,20,21] This implies that there are two distinct varieties of CCK receptors, one located in the periphery, which is selective for sulphated CCK, and the other located in the central nervous system that is selective for nonsulphated CCK. These have been termed the peripheral or alimentary CCK A or 1 receptor and the central or brain CCK B or 2 receptor.[22,23]

SYNTHESIS AND DEGRADATION OF CHOLECYSTOKININ

Cloning and sequence analysis of a cDNA encoding preprocholecystokinin from rat thyroid carcinoma, porcine brain, and porcine intestine reveals 345 nucleotides coding for a precursor to CCK, which is 115 amino acids and contains all the cholecystokinin sequences previously isolated.[24,25,26]

Synthesis and degradation from the prepro-CCK is by posttranslational processing steps including sulphation of the tyrosines, cleavage of the C-terminal Gly-Arg-Arg extension, amidation of the C-terminal phenylalanine, cleavage of the *N*-terminal leader sequence, cleavage of the carboxyl side of Arg-74 of pro-CCK,[27] and cleavages to CCK-58 and smaller peptides.[28] Enzymes involved in posttranslational processing include a 34,000 molecular weight intestinal enzyme that appears to be a nontrypsin protease that degrades CCK-33 to CCK-12.[26] Degradation of sulphated CCK octapeptides to inactive fragments may occur through a membrane-bound aminopeptidase that cleaves sulphated CCK-8, unsulphated CCK-8, and CCK-4.[29] Enkephalinase, a membrane-bound neutral metalloendopeptidase that also degrades the peptides enkephalin, angiotensin, substance P, and neurotensin, cleaves CCK-8 at the Gly^4-Trp^5 bond, the Trp^5-Met^6 bond and the Asp^7-Phe^8 bond.[30,31]

Chapter 4

Cholecystokinin As a Gut Peptide

Although the major focus of our attention is on the relationship between CCK and pain and hence the more central role of CCK, this peptide also serves important gastrointestinal functions. CCK is found in the duodenum and jejunum[1,2] with a small amount in the ileum.[2] CCK is also found in enteric nerves.[3] CCK-like immunoreactivity is detectable in human plasma at levels of around 1 pmol^{-1}.[4] Immunochemical studies have confirmed that CCK is synthesized by the mucosal endocrine I cells[5,6] and to a certain extent by the duodenal cells that resemble K cells of the small intestine and A cells of the pancreas.[7]

CHOLECYSTOKININ RELEASE

In healthy volunteers, ingestion of fat and protein, but not starch, causes a significant increase in plasma CCK levels.[8] In humans, plasma CCK concentrations are consistently elevated by fatty acids with a chain of 12 carbon atoms or longer, whereas those of 11 or fewer carbon atoms fail to increase CCK levels.[9] Of the amino acids, phenylalanine is the most potent stimulant of CCK release.[10,11] Carbohydrate and glucose appear to be weak stimulants of CCK release.[8,12,13] Instillation of hydrochloric acid has been shown to cause a marked increase in CCK release in humans,[14] dogs,[15] and in pigs.[16] When less concentrated acid is used, the increase in CCK levels in humans is lessened.[17] Therefore, the contribution of hydrochloric acid under physiological conditions may not be significant.

Cholecystokinin and Its Antagonists in Pain Management

doi:10.1300/5593_04

EFFECT OF CCK

Ivy and Oldberg's (1928) work pointed out that CCK has an effect on gallbladder function. In humans, after eating, there is a decrease in gallbladder volume.[18] Similarly, when CCK is administered intravenously to achieve the plasma concentrations seen after feeding, a similar decrease in gallbladder volume is observed.[18] If CCK A antagonists are administered and then CCK intravenously infused, then no decrease in gallbladder is observed.[19,20] Similarly, the decreases in gallbladder volume observed after eating are also blocked by CCK A antagonists.[19-21]

When pancreatic exocrine function in humans is considered, CCK A receptors are found on pancreatic acinar cells.[22-25] Treatments known to increase endogenous CCK levels also increase pancreatic exocrine secretion[26-29] while interventions that return CCK levels to basal levels decrease pancreatic exocrine secretion.[30] A CCK antagonist or atropine completely blocks the effect of exogenous CCK on pancreatic exocrine secretion,[31,32] while it only partially blocks the effect of increased endogenous CCK.[21,31-33] It seems that in humans, CCK and the cholinergic system act together in the regulation of pancreatic enzyme secretion.

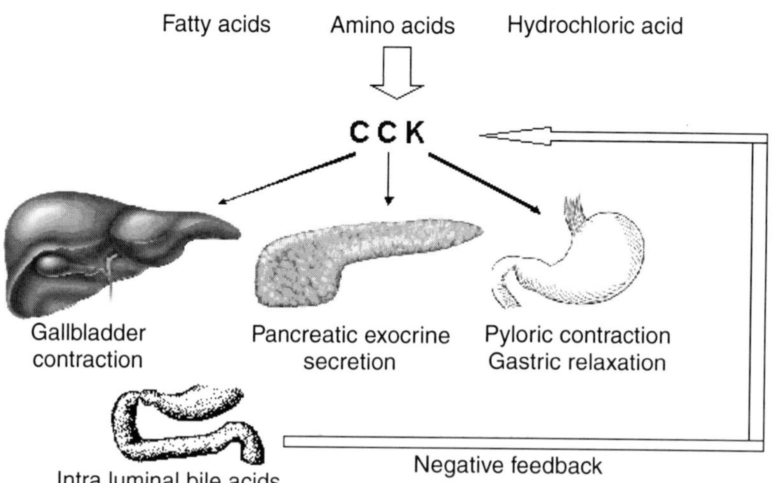

FIGURE 4.1. Stimulation of endogenous CCK release, target organ effects, and inhibition of release by bile acids.

Exogenous CCK contracts the pyloric sphincter and relaxes the proximal stomach with consequent slowing of gastric emptying in rats, nonhuman primates, and humans.[34-37] It is likely that vagal afferents are important in this effect as an intact gastric branch of the vagus nerve is required for this action.[38,39] When a CCK A antagonist is administered to mice or rats, any rise in CCK produced by a mixed test meal is not associated with any slowing of gastric emptying.[40] However, in humans, CCK A antagonists have no effect on the response to a test meal in doses that significantly inhibit postprandial gallbladder emptying (see Figure 4.1).[21,40-42]

A variety of stimuli lead to an increase in endogenous CCK levels with consequent effects on the gallbladder, exocrine pancreatic secretion, and gastric emptying. When bile enters the duodenum it causes a reflex decrease in CCK release, whether this release is postprandial or stimulated by other factors[43-46] and this decrease in CCK release cannot be further inhibited by exogenous bile acid administration.[47] Overall, bile acids are the most important luminal regulators of CCK release in humans.[47]

Chapter 5

Cholecystokinin As a Central Nervous System Peptide

In 1975 Vanderhaegen and colleagues described, for the first time, the presence of CCK in the central nervous system.[1] This finding was soon after confirmed by Dockray (1976).[2] Within a few years others had shown the presence of CCK in the central nervous system of rats, guinea pigs,[3] pigs,[4] and humans.[5]

A number of investigational techniques have been used to study the presence and distribution of CCK in the central nervous system. These studies are hindered by the fact that in vivo, systemically administered peptides do not cross the blood-brain barrier. Initial investigations utilized immunochemical and radioimmunochemical techniques. Larsson and Renfeld showed that CCK-containing nerves were particularly numerous in the neocortex, hippocampus, amygdaloid nuclei, hypothalamus, and spinal cord of the guinea pig.[6] Ju and colleagues (1987) found that in the spinal cord of the rat, CCK-like immunoreactivity was present in the spinothalamic neurons, whose cell bodies were located in the lumbar segments L1-L5 with preferential localization dorsal to the central canal at rostral levels and lateral to the canal at caudal levels. These cells projected via the ventral part of the lateral funiculus to the most ventral and posterior parts of the thalamus. Here, they found a distinct, varicose terminal network which extended caudally from an area lateral to the medial lemniscus, running medially over the medial lemniscus, traversing the parafasicular nucleus, and running dorsal to the fasciculus retroflexus into the periventricular gray matter.[7]

CCK A AND CCK B

With the advent of CCK antagonists, both CCK A and CCK B, further elucidation of the central distribution of CCK was possible. These nonpeptides could be used to allow differentiation between CCK A and CCK B receptors and their relative distribution in the nervous system. If a radiolabelled CCK fragment is administered, its presence can be detected, for example, using autoradiography. If a specific CCK antagonist is administered, the displacement of the radiolabelled CCK fragment allows conclusion of the type of CCK receptor that fragment occupied.

Using these techniques, Hill and Woodruff (1990) showed that in rat and monkey brains, ^{125}I-BH-CCK binding was localized regionally with high levels being detected in the cerebral cortex, basal ganglia, and some mid- and hind-brain nuclei. Specific binding was also localized to the substantia gelatinosa of the rat, monkey, and human spinal cord. The CCK B antagonist, L365,260 inhibited binding to most areas of the brain except in the rat medial nucleus tractus solitarii and the monkey nucleus tractus solitarii, dorsomedial nucleus and infundibular hypothalamic nuclei together with the dorsomedial aspects of the caudate nucleus where CCK Λ sites were present. In the primate spinal cord, L365,260 was a relatively weak inhibitor of ^{125}I-BH-CCK binding, whereas the CCK A antagonist MK-329 showed high affinity for the CCK A sites present there. In contrast, in the rat, L365,260 showed higher affinity than MK-329 for the binding sites in the dorsal horn indicating a species difference in the distribution of the subtypes of CCK receptors.[8]

DISTRIBUTION OF CCK RECEPTORS

Many studies in murine and rodent models showed a preponderance of CCK B receptors in the central nervous system, with CCK A being in preponderance in the alimentary tract (hence Moran's classification of CCK A (alimentary), B (brain). In the few studies of primates, a different picture emerged. For example, in the study by Hill and colleagues (1990), using a primate model (cynomolgus monkey), the use of radiolabeled CCK and radiolabeled CCK antagonist were used to study the distribution of CCK. They defined CCK A receptors, in this case, as those which displayed a high affinity for the selective

CCK A antagonist MK-329 as evidenced by its selective inhibition of ^{125}I-BH-CCK or by direct labeling with ^{3}H-MK-329. In this primate model, high densities of CCK A sites were found in the nucleus tractus solitarius and also in the dorsal motor nucleus of the vagus. In addition, CCK A sites were localized to a number of hypothalamic nuclei such as the supraoptic and paraventricular nuclei, the dorso-medial and infundibular nuclei, as well as the neurohypophysis. The mammilary bodies and supramammiliary nuclei also contained CCK A receptor sites. High concentrations of CCK A receptors were present in the substantia nigra zona compacta and also the ventral tegmental area.[9] The extensive representation of CCK A and its binding sites in the primate CNS is in marked contrast to the preponderance of the B variety in other species.

Another method used in determining the distribution of CCK in the nervous system revolves around the detection of cells containing mRNA encoding CCK. A complementary DNA (cDNA) clone for CCK mRNA was first isolated from rat by Deschenes and colleagues (1984).[10] Both human and rat CCK mRNA encode a 115 amino acid CCK prepropeptide. Regional distribution of preproCCK mRNA, usually denoted as CCK mRNA for simplicity, has been studied using in situ hybridization and Northern blot analysis. In the human brain, the highest CCK mRNA levels are detected in the neocortex, lower levels in the amygdaloid complex, and even lower levels in the thalamus.[11] Lindefors and colleagues (1993) examined brain tissue of individuals who had died of acute coronary insufficiency. They demonstrated CCK mRNA in the neocortex and hippocampus but could detect no CCK mRNA in the thalamus. In one individual, evidence of the presence of CCK was found in the substantia nigra. Variable levels were also found in the claustrum.[12]

When in situ hybridization techniques are used to detect cells containing mRNA-encoding cholecystokinin, these cells are considerably more numerous than when immunochemical techniques are used. It seems that in situ hybridization is more sensitive than the immunochemical methods at detecting these cells. In some brain areas, CCK mRNA is easily detectable and yet immunoreactivity for CCK is entirely absent.[13] The definitive reasons for this need clarification.

Cholecystokinin-mRNA-containing neurons are numerous in the central nervous system. In studies on rats, Schiffmann and Vanderhaegen (1991) found that neurons expressing mRNA for CCK were found in the olfactory bulb, olfactory nuclei, layers II-III and V-VI of the cerebral cortex, amygdaloid nuclei, subiculum, hippocampus, claustrum, endopiriform nucleus, several hypothalamic nuclei, most of the thalamic nuclei, ventral tegmental area, substantia nigra, interfascicularis nucleus, linearis rostralis, central gray, Edinger-Westphal nucleus, superior and inferior colliculi, parabrachial nucleus, reticular formation, raphe nuclei, and spinal trigeminal nucleus.[13] They also showed that several brain areas such as the thalamus and colliculi contained CCK mRNA but were devoid of perikarya exhibiting CCK-like immunoreactivity. Furthermore, they found that the cerebral cortex and hippocampus displayed a far higher density of CCK mRNA containing cells than perikarya containing CCK-like immunoreactivity.

Despite the differences in CCK content detected using different experimental techniques and the obvious species differences in the type of CCK subtypes, it is very clear that CCK is widely distributed in the central nervous system. In the forthcoming chapters we will see that this widespread distribution is matched by an importance in modulating a number of neural systems, and in particular those related to pain perception.

Chapter 6

Central Effect of Cholecystokinin

In the previous chapter, the extensive central representation of CCK was discussed. In forthcoming chapters, the relevance of CCK in terms of nociception will be considered. In this section, some insight into the neurochemical and neurophysiological actions of CCK will be considered.

OPIOID RECEPTORS AND INTRACELLULAR CALCIUM

In 1989 Wang and colleagues showed that CCK-8 inhibited the high affinity binding for [^{3}H]etorphine, a universal ligand for mu, delta, and kappa opioid receptors.[1]

In order to refine this knowledge and try to elucidate that CCK has a specific effect on an individual type of opioid receptor, Wand and Han (1990) utilized more specific radiolabeled opioid receptor ligands. For mu receptors they used [tyrosly-3,5-^{3}H][D-Ala^2,MePhe^4, Gly-ol^5]enkephalin ([^{3}H]DAGO), for the delta receptor [tyrosol-3,5-^{3}H][D-Pen^{2,5}]enkephalin ([^{3}H]DPDPE) and [^{3}H]U69,593 for the kappa receptor. They found that CCK-8 inhibited binding of mu and kappa, but not delta receptors. They further observed that CCK-8 suppressed the affinity for kappa receptors and reduced the number of mu receptors.[2]

Zhang and colleagues (2000) used single and double-color immunofluorescence to study the relationship between mu opioid receptors and CCK-like immunoreactivity in superficial dorsal horn neurons. They found that fibers containing mu opioid receptor and CCK-like immunoreactivity were found in laminae I and II. Mu opioid receptor-like immunoreactivity was present in 65 percent of counted CCK-positive neuron profiles.[3] Most CCK-positive neuron profiles contained mu opioid receptors.[4] There is a considerable co-localization of CCK-like immunoreactivity and mu opioid-like immunoreactivity in lamina II dorsal horn neurons. This suggests that these CCK-containing neurons may be directly activated by opioids since they also contain mu opioid receptors and that administration of an opioid may cause release of CCK. Since there are also other CCK-positive neurons in lamina II of the dorsal horn, which do not exhibit CCK-like immunoreactivity, it is possible that these neurons release CCK in response to stimuli other than morphine such as potassium.

Although CCK may inhibit binding of specific opioid ligands to receptors, its effect may also be postreceptor. In isolated rat pancreatic acinar cells CCK-8 causes an increase in cytoplasmic calcium concentration, the calcium being mobilized from internal cellular calcium stores.[5] Wang and colleagues (1992) reported that in enzymatically dissociated brain cells prepared from neonatal rats, KCl induced a significant increase in free intracellular calcium ions and this increase could be blocked by agents which block voltage-gated calcium channels. The opioid receptor agonists OMF (mu receptor specific), DPDPE (delta), and 66A-078 (kappa) showed a highly significant suppressive effect on Ca^{2+} influx induced by high K^+ depolarization. CCK-8 dose-dependently mobilized Ca^{2+} from intracellular stores. CCK-8 did not affect significantly the increase in free intracellular Ca^{2+} following high K^+. However, it did reverse the opioid suppression of high K^+ induced increase in free intracellular Ca^{2+} by the mu and kappa agonists.[6] This finding, an effect on calcium mobilization by CCK-8 when related to stimulation of the mu and kappa, but not delta opioid receptors, is similar to the effect of CCK-8 on binding of opioid ligands to these receptors.

When morphine is administered systemically, an induced dose-dependent and naloxone-reversible increase of the release of CCK-like immunoreactivity occurs. When the L-type calcium channel blocker verapamil or the n-type calcium channel blocker omega-conotoxin are applied topically onto the dorsal horn, the release of CCK-like immunoreactivity induced by morphine is completely blocked.[7]

Due to the discovery of the mu, delta, and kappa opioid receptors, it is now known that another opioid receptor, the orphan or ORL1 receptor, also exists. Its functions differ and even oppose those of the other opioid receptors. The hecta-peptide, orphanin FQ/nociceptin

("nociceptin") is an endogenous ligand of the ORL1 receptor. Supraspinally, it causes antiopioid effects[8,9] while at the spinal level it causes analgesia.[10-12] In contrast to the effect of other opioid ligands, the inhibitory effect of nociceptin in neuropathic rats is enhanced by CCK,[13] emphasizing the difference between the ORL1 and other opioid receptors.

NORADRENALINE RELEASE IN THE RAT SUPRAOPTIC NUCLEUS

Systemic administration of CCK results in the expression of Fos-like immunoreactivity in many neurones of the nucleus tractus solitarius. Fos is the protein product of the immediate-early gene c-Fos whose expression is induced in many neuronal systems following afferent-induced activation. The expression of Fos in A2 neurones of the supraoptic nucleus following CCK administration suggests that this cell group is the origin of the noradrenaline release observed in the supraoptic nucleus in response to CCK.[14,15] Onaka and colleagues (1995) have shown that systemic administration of CCK blocked CCK-induced Fos expression in supraoptic neurones but had no effect on Fos-like protein induction in C2/A2 catecholaminergic neurones.[14]

DYNORPHIN

When dynorphin is administered in small amounts it has an anti-analgesic action against morphine.[15,16,17] This effect appears to be indirect and requires involvement of an ascending pathway to the brain and a descending pathway to the spinal cord. Rady and colleagues (1999) have shown that morphine analgesia was inhibited by dynorphin as shown by a rightward shift of the morphine dose-response curve. The effect of dynorphin was eliminated by administration of the CCK antagonists lorglumide and PD135 158. Pretreatment with CCK antiserum also eliminated the effect of dynorphin. On the other hand, the antianalgesic action of CCK was not affected by dynorphin antiserum. They concluded that the antianalgesic action of dynorphin occurred through an indirect mechanism ultimately dependent on the action of spinal CCK.[18]

DELTA OPIOID RECEPTORS

The antinociceptive potency of morphine is altered by the presence of agonists of the delta opioid receptor. [Leu[5]]enkephalin, an endogenous ligand of the delta opioid receptor increases the antinociceptive potency of intracerebroventricular morphine in the mouse.[19-21]

Vanderah and colleagues (1994) have investigated the effect of delta opioid receptor ligands on morphine-induced antinociception. They utilized a synthetic oligodeoxynucleotide (oligo) complementary to the 5' coding region of the cloned mouse CCK B receptor (antisense), a mismatch oligo. Intracerebroventricular (i.c.v.) treatment of mice with CCK B antisense for three days resulted in an enhancement of the antinociceptive potency of i.c.v. morphine as indicated by a sixfold shift to the left of the dose-response curve. When they investigated the antinociceptive effect of morphine in control animals, CCK B antisense-treated animals in the presence and absence of naltrindole (a delta opioid receptor antagonist) as well as in the presence or absence of antisera directed against [Leu[5]]- or [Met[5]]enkephalin, they found that the enhanced potency of morphine in mice pretreated with CCK B antisense oligo was blocked by naltrindole and antisera to [Leu[5]] enkephalin, but not [Met[5]] enkephalin. Naltrindole or antisera toward [Leu[5]]enkephalin or [Met[5]]enkephalin did not produce antinociceptive effects when given alone. They suggest that CCK may act via CCK B receptors (in the mouse) to tonically inhibit the release of [Leu[5]]enkephalin or a [Leu[5]]enkephalin-like peptide and that the enhancement of morphine antinociception seen in the presence of CCK B receptor blockade may be the result of the enhancement of morphine antinociception by delta opioid receptors.[22,23]

ROSTRAL VENTROMEDIAL MEDULLA

Three physiologically distinct populations of neurones have been identified in the rostro ventromedial medulla (RVM). (1) OFF cells activated by mu opioid agonists,[24,25] (2) ON cells that display a sudden increase in activity just before the occurrence of a nocifensive reflex and which exert a facilitating effect on nociception and are directly inhibited by mu opioid agonists,[26,27] and (3) neutral cells that show no change in activity associated with nociceptive responses and do not respond to opioid administration.[28] Heinricher and colleagues

(2001) found that direct injection of CCK into the RVM by itself had no effect on tail-flick latency or on the firing of any cell class measured, but significantly attenuated opioid activation of OFF cells and inhibited its effect on the tail-flick test. Opioid suppression of ON-cell firing was not significantly altered by CCK.[29] This shows that CCK acting within the RVM attenuates the analgesic effect of morphine by preventing activation of the pain inhibiting output neurones of the RVM, the OFF cells.

DOPAMINE

Dopamine has been found to be colocalized in the ventral tegmental area and substantia nigra with CCK.[30,31] Infusion of CCK into the nucleus accumbens has effects on dopamine release. If infused into the shell of this nucleus, then dopamine release is increased while infusion into the core causes a decreased release.[32-34] If CCK is infused into the ventral tegmental area, then dopamine is released into the nucleus accumbens and amygdala.[35] Although it has not been suggested that the action of CCK on dopamine release has direct effects on nociception, there may be a clearer link between CCK-induced dopamine release and certain behavior traits.[36]

ALPHA ADRENERGIC RECEPTORS

The dorsal horn of the spinal cord is known to be an important site for the antinociceptive effects of opioids. Similarly, it is of importance in the antinociceptive effects of alpha adrenergic agonists such as clonidine and dexmedetomidine.[37-39] Sullivan and colleagues (1994) measured extracellular recordings of noxious-evoked C fiber responses of dorsal horn neurones in anesthetized rats. When given alone, the alpha 2 adrenergic agonist dexmedetomidine significantly reduced C fiber-evoked responses. When dexmedetomidine was given in the presence of CCK, the profound reduction in the C fiber-evoked response was significantly attenuated. When selective CCK B receptor antagonists were given with the alpha adrenoreceptor agonist, evoked responses were not altered.[40] This suggests that CCK is able to inhibit spinal antinociception mediated by the activation of

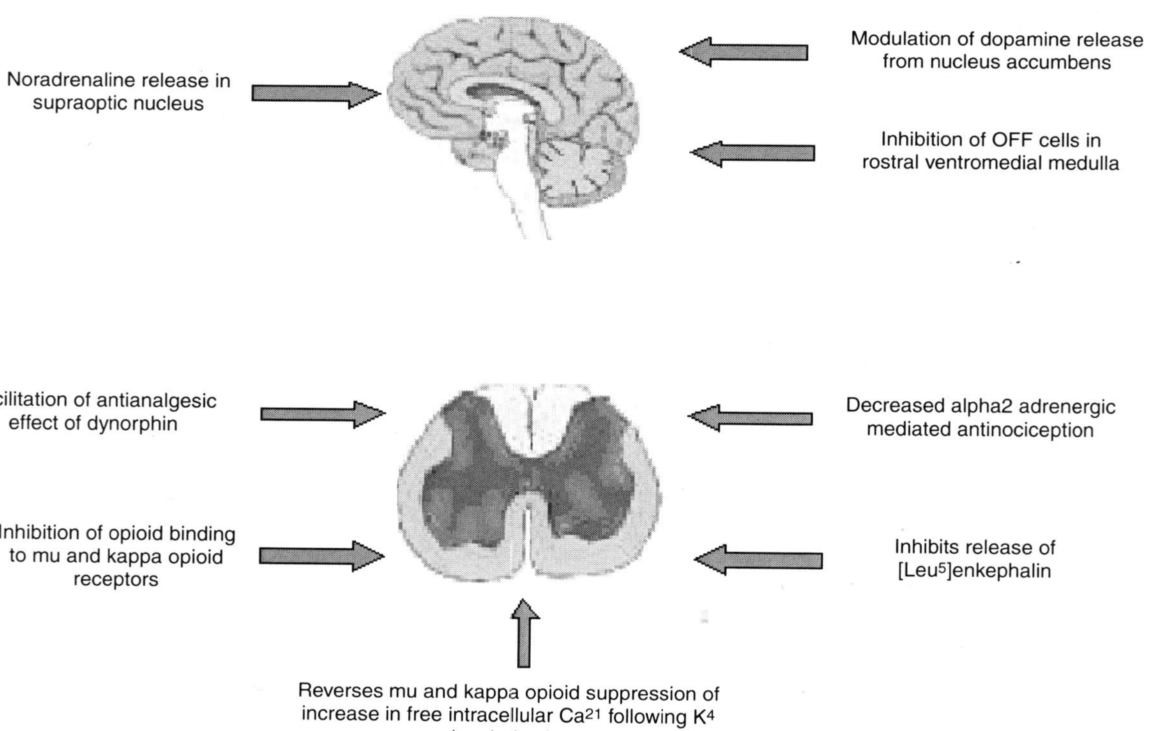

FIGURE 6.1. Postulated effects of cholecystokinin in the central nervous system.

34

alpha 2 adrenergic receptors but that CCK antagonists do not influence this alpha-adrenergic-receptor-mediated antinociception.

Clearly, CCK is widely distributed in the CNS and it is linked to many areas of the CNS which are known to be of importance in nociceptive processing (see Figure 6.1). The relative importance of each individual location where CCK is found and its actions at these sites is open to debate: in combination, the importance is beyond debate.

In forthcoming chapters, we will see how the level of CCK in the CNS is influenced by a number of factors, important in patients with pain, and how these alterations in CCK levels can have an adverse effect on pain perception.

Chapter 7

Factors That Increase Central Cholecystokinin Representation

CCK is colocalized in the gut and central nervous system. It seems to be found in particular association wih the opioid receptors, and, as we will later see, has an important effect on opioid-derived analgesia.

Given this importance, any factors that could influence the extent of its central representation could have important implications for the quality of analgesia derived from the use of opioids. In this chapter, we will review the major influences on the representation of CCK in the CNS.

POTASSIUM

The effect of K^+ on extracellular CCK levels has been investigated using microdialysis techniques and radioimmunoassay for determining CCK levels.[1] The tip of the dialysis probe is placed between laminae VI and VII to ensure that the CCK that is collected originates primarily in the dorsal spinal cord. Using this technique, Wiesenfeld-Hallin and colleagues (1999) found that the basal level of CCK in normal rats as about the lowest level detectable by the radioimmunoassay technique. Increases of K^+ by 25 or 50mM for 30 minutes failed to induce any significant rise in CCK-like immunoreactivity. However, when the probe was perfused with Krebs-Ringer solution to increase the K^+ concentration to 100mM then a sixfold increase in the extracellular CCK-like immunoreactivity was detected.[2] In contrast, such increases in K^+ in axotomized rats induced no significant increase in extracellular CCK.[2] When a CCK antagonist is administered along with a perfusion to achieve an increase in K^+ in axotomized rats, then CCK levels do increase. It has been suggested that axotomy induces changes in the mechanisms of CCK release induced by membrane depolarization and that the response to coadministration of a CCK antagonist implies that CCK is present in axotomized rats. Since alteration of K^+ concentration has an effect on Ca^{2+} channels, then in axotomized animals, a malfunction of the K^+/Ca^{2+} channels in certain groups of neurones following nerve section may lead to reduced CCK exocytosis.

NEURAL INJURY

Xu and colleagues (1993) studied the effect of unilateral spinal nerve ligation on the expression of CCK mRNA. When control animals were examined, only a few dorsal root ganglia were found to be CCK mRNA positive. Similarly, the sides contralateral to the sides of injury were examined in nerve-ligated animals; few CCK mRNA positive cells were observed. In contrast, fourteen days after axotomy, up to 30 percent of all ganglia cells were positive in axotomized animals on the side of injury.[3] This lack of CCK mRNA in uninjured rat primary sensory neurones is a consistent finding[4,5,6] while the presence of CCK mRNA in around 30 percent of dorsal root ganglia cells in axotomized animals is again a consistent finding.[7]

Zhang and colleagues (1993) have shown that mRNA for the CCK B receptor is present at very low levels in normal dorsal root ganglia of the rat, but that axotomy causes a very marked increase in the number of sensory neurones expressing CCK B receptor mRNA.[8] Therefore, it is both the mRNA for CCK and its receptor that are increased by axotomy, at least in the rat.

Verge and colleagues (1993) investigated the presence of CCK mRNA in a primate (monkey) model and compared it to that found in the rat. They confirmed the findings of others that CCK mRNA is virtually undetectable in the rat dorsal root ganglia cell in the absence of axotomy and its presence in around 30 percent of ganglia cells after axotomy. In contrast, they found that CCK mRNA was detectable in around 20 percent of monkey dorsal root ganglion neurones, regardless of spinal level, in the absence of neural injury. Furthermore, they found that 10 percent of trigeminal ganglia neurones also expressed CCK mRNA. They also found that in the monkey spinal cord, CCK mRNA was detectable in the dorsal horn and in the motoneurons.[7]

As with the dorsal root ganglion neurones, those in the dorsal horn of the rat do not express CCK mRNA in any quantity. Similarly, it is normally not possible to detect CCK-like immunoreactivity in rodent primary afferent neurones.[9] As with dorsal root ganglia neurones, when a microdialysis probe is perfused with K+ (100mM), there is a sixfold increase in the extracellular level of CCK-like immunoreactivity in control animals. After axotomy, no such increase in CCK-like immunoreactivity occurs after K+ perfusion, unless the animal is pretreated with a specific CCK antagonist.[10]

Bras and colleagues (1999) also investigated the effect of peripheral axotomy on CCK expression. They found that 14 days after axotomy there was a 70 percent increase in the CCK B receptor mRNA levels on the side of the axotomy as well as a very marked increase in the autoradiographic labeling of CCK B receptors by the tritiated CCK B agonist [3H]pBC 264. However, measurement of dorsal root ganglia at L4-L6 levels revealed no significant changes in proCCK mRNA after nerve lessioning.[11] They suggested that up-regulation of CCK B receptors, rather than CCK synthesis and release, seemed to be demonstrated.

When spinal injuries are inflicted on experimental animals, only a proportion exhibit features of neuropathic pain. To investigate the relationship between spinal nerve injury and the presence of neuropathic pain, Xu and colleagues (2001) examined the cerebrospinal fluid (CSF) of spinally injured and control rats. They found a basal level of CCK-like immunoreactivity present in the CSF of control rats. In spinally injured rats that did not exhibit evidence of allodynia (as measured by assessing vocalization thresholds using von Frey filaments), levels of CCK-like immunoreactivity were around those found in uninjured animals. However, in those spinally injured rats who exhibited features of allodynia, a threefold increase in CSF CCK-like immunoreactivity was detected[12] (Figure 7.1).

GAMMA-AMINOBUTYRIC ACID

CCK-like immunoreactivity is reduced after stimulation by gamma-aminobutyric acid (GABA) and its related agonists in the cerebral cortex,[13] neostriatum,[14] and spinal cord[15] in vitro. Both GABA-A and

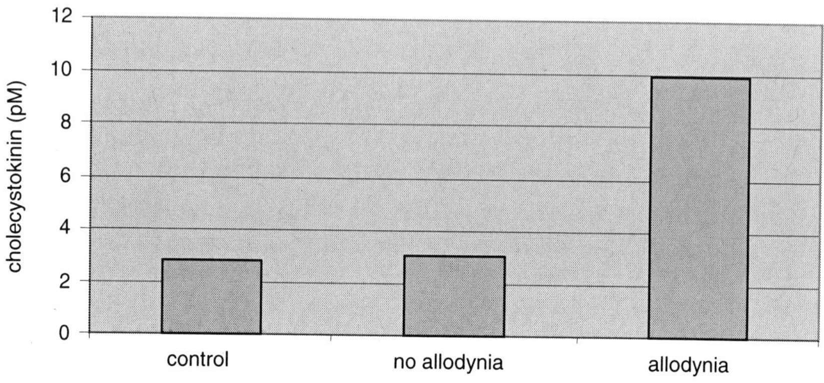

FIGURE 7.1. Average concentration of CCK-like immunoreactivity in CSF from normal (n = 8), spinally injured nonallodynic (n = 8), and allodynic rats (n = 9). (*Source:* Reprinted from *Peptides,* 22, Xu X-J, Alster P, Wu W-P, Hao J-X, Wiesenfeld-Hallin Z. Increased level of cholecystokinin in cerebrospinal fluid is associated with chronic pain-like behaviour in spinally injured rats, pp. 1305-1308, copyright 2001, with permission from Elsevier.)

GABA-B agonists reduce CCK release.[16] It is possible, therefore, that at least a proportion of the antinociceptive effect of GABA agonists is related to their ability to reduce spinal CCK release.

VASOACTIVE INTESTINAL PEPTIDE

Vasoactive intestinal peptide (VIP) can modulate the K^+ induced release of CCK-like immunoreactivity. In the caudate-putamen, K^+ evoked release of CCK-like immunoreactivity is inhibited by low doses of VIP.[17] Conversely, VIP does not inhibit CCK release from the cerebral cortex.[18] In the spinal cord, CCK and VIP are released by K^+ depolarization in a calcium-dependent manner[19] and it is possible that VIP has an influence on the release of CCK in spinal cord dorsal horn neurones. After peripheral axotomy, VIP is upregulated in the dorsal root ganglia[20,21] and this could contribute to decreased release of CCK from the spinal cord following peripheral axotomy.

MORPHINE

In 1993 Zhou and colleagues were the first to show that systemic morphine produced a marked increase in CCK-8 immunoreactivity in the perfusate of rat spinal cord and that this effect was completely reversed by the administration of naloxone[22] (Figure 7.2). Ding and Bayer (1993) assessed the effects of single and repeated administration of morphine on both CCK mRNA and CCK in different brain areas and the spinal cord. They found that a single injection of morphine resulted in a significant increase in CCK mRNA content in the hypothalamus and spinal cord. No changes in CCK peptide concentrations were observed in any of the brain areas they examined. After repeated injections of morphine, the rats became completely tolerant to the analgesic effects of the morphine. At the same time, increases in CCK mRNA and CCK peptide were observed in the hypothala-

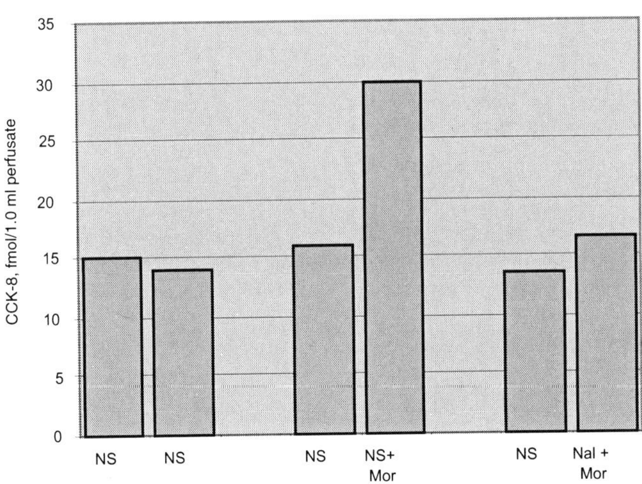

FIGURE 7.2. The increase in CCK-8 immunoreactivity in the spinal perfusate elicited by systemic morphine and its blockade by intrathecal naloxone. Normal saline administered followed after ten minutes by normal saline, morphine or morphine and naloxone (NS = normal saline, Mor = morphine, Nal = naloxone). (*Source:* Reprinted from *European Journal of Pharmacology,* 234, Zhou Y, Sun Y-H, Zhang Z-W, Han J-S. Increased release of immunoreactive cholecystokinin octapeptide by morphine and potentiation of mu-opioid analgesia by CCK B receptor antagonist L-365,260 in rat spinal cord, pp. 147-154, copyright 1993, with permission from Elsevier.)

mus, spinal cords, and brainstem. They suggested that the differing levels of CCK peptide found with acute and chronic treatment with morphine implied that repeated opioid administration results in an increased endogenous CCK peptide content due to an increased rate of CCK biosynthesis in the central nervous system.[23] This increase in CCK immunoreactivity may have resulted from an increase not only of synthesis of CCK in the spinal cord, hypothalamus, and brainstem, but also from an increased release from nerve terminals of neurones projecting to these regions.

In animals, spinal morphine has an increased potency in those with carrageenin-induced inflammation. Stanfa and Dickenson (1993) studied the effect of morphine treatment on the C-fiber-evoked responses of single dorsal horn nociceptive neurones. In the presence of carrageenin-induced inflammation, morphine significantly reduced C-fiber-evoked responses when compared to control animals. When the animals were pretreated with the specific CCK B receptor antagonist, L365,260, in control animals the effect of morphine administration in reducing C-fiber-evoked responses was increased. However, in those animals with carrageenin-induced inflammation, there was no alteration in the response to morphine. When CCK was administered, CCK attenuated the effect of morphine only in animals with carrageenin-induced inflammation, having no effect on normal animals. They suggested that morphine produced a maximal release of CCK in normal animals which could not be further enhanced by exogenous CCK administration.[24]

Zhang and colleagues (2000) examined the effects on mu-opioid receptor and CCK-receptor immunoreactivity in rat spinal dorsal horn neurones after peripheral axotomy and inflammation. They found that mu-opioid receptor-like immunoreactivity was present in 65 percent of CCK-positive neurones in lamina I and II of the spinal cord. Conversely, 40 percent of mu-opioid receptor-positive neurones contained CCK-like immunoreactivity. When morphine was administered after sciatic nerve section, there was a significant reduction in mu-opioid receptor-like immunoreactivity in the medial half of lamina II in the L5 segment of the ipsilateral dorsal horn, with a similar reduction in CCK-like immunoreactivity. These changes could be prevented by naloxone pretreatment. No such changes were seen in animals with induced inflammation.[25] There were no changes on mu-opioid-receptor distribution in lamina I in axotomized animals treated with morphine. The decrease in mu-opioid receptor-like immuno-reactivity observed in the superficial dorsal horn ipsilateral to the nerve injury was observed within thirty minutes and did not recover, suggesting that release of CCK took place and that this release may be related to activation of opioid receptors and to the decrease in mu-opioid receptor-like immunoreactivity observed.

Once again, the clear relationship between CCK, CCK receptors, and the opioidergic systems has been highlighted. Very definite changes in the presence of CCK-like immunoreactivity follow peripheral axotomy and morphine administration. These are matched by changes in concentrations of free CSF CCK. In the following chapters, the relevance of these changes will become apparent.

Chapter 8

Cholecystokinin
As an Antiopioid Peptide

The importance of CCK revolves around its effect on opioid-derived antinociception. The evidence for this effect is twofold. First, exogenously administered CCK has a pro-nociceptive effect, and second, CCK antagonists can enhance the antinociceptive effect of opioids. This latter effect will be examined in a later chapter. In this section we will consider the effect of exogenous CCK on nociception.

EFFECT OF CCK
ON OPIOID ANTINOCICEPTION

When a brief electrical shock is applied to the rat front paw on a regular basis, a so-called unconditioned stimulus, opiate-type analgesia, is produced.[1] Faris and colleagues (1983) studied rats with this front-paw-shock-induced analgesia. Analgesia was assessed using a tail-flick test. CCK-8 or saline was injected intraperitoneally. Tail latency was assessed before and at regular intervals after exposure to the shock. They found that all but the lowest dose of CCK-8 significantly reduced front-paw-shock-induced analgesia[2] (Figure 8.1). This front-paw-shock-induced analgesia was antagonized by naloxone administration.[3]

In another experiment, Faris and colleagues (1983) injected rats intraperitoneally with morphine 20 minutes after giving them either saline or CCK-8. Tail-flick latencies were then measured. In those animals pretreated with CCK-8, administration of morphine had significantly less effect than in those in which saline was used, showing that CCK-8 antagonized the effect of morphine[2] (Figure 8.2).

When CCK is injected into rat paws inflamed with Freund's adjuvant, it produces no antinociceptive effect. When the mu-opioid

Cholecystokinin and Its Antagonists in Pain Management
© 2006 by The Haworth Press, Inc. All rights reserved.
doi:10.1300/5593_08

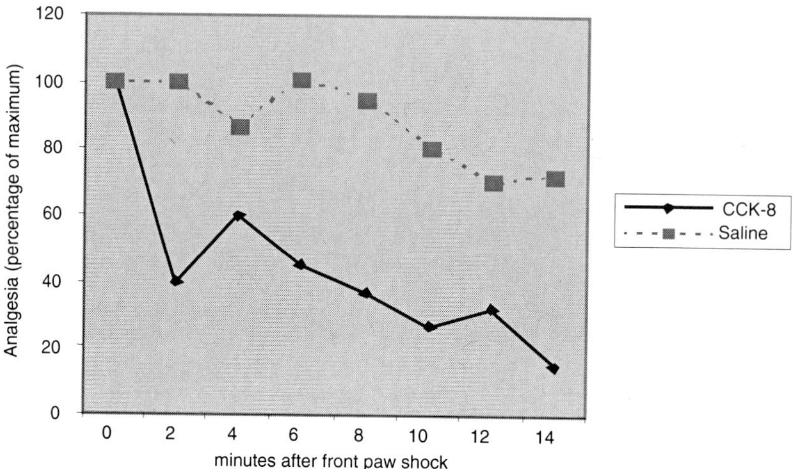

FIGURE 8.1. Reduction in front-paw-shock-induced analgesia caused by intraperitoneal CCK-8 compared with saline. (*Source:* Reprinted with permission from Faris PL, Komisaruk BR, Watkins LR, Mayer DJ. Evidence for the neuropeptide cholecystokinin as an antagonist of opiate analgesia. *Science* 1983; 219: 310-312. Copyright 1983, AAAS.)

receptor agonists [D-Ala[2],N-methyl-Phe[4],Gly-ol[5]]-enkephalin or fentanyl are administered parenterally, an antinociceptive effect is observed. However, if CCK is injected into the inflamed paw along with parenteral mu-opioid agonist, the antinociceptive effect of the opioid is attenuated.[4] Note that this study utilized doses of 0.1 and 1 µg of CCK. Later studies used substantially larger doses of CCK and produced results that suggest an antinociceptive effect of CCK. It could be argued that these larger doses were "pharmacological" rather than the "physiological" dose used in this study.

INFLUENCE OF CCK TYPE
ON OPIOID ANTINOCICEPTION

The effect of CCK may not be related only to the dose administered, but also to the form of CCK which is either exogenously administered or endogenously raised. When a mixed CCK A & B analogue [Boc-Tyr(SO$_3$H)-Nle-Gly-Trp-Nle-Asp-Phe-NH$_2$] is administered to rats, the rat-jump latency is increased and this effect is

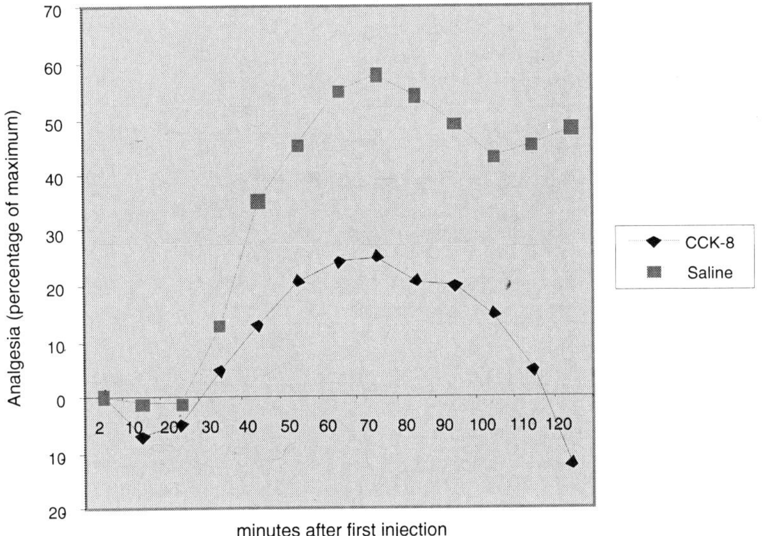

FIGURE 8.2. Antagonism of morphine-induced analgesia by CCK-8. CCK-8 or saline injected at T = 0 followed at T = 20 by morphine. (*Source:* Reprinted with permission from Faris PL, Komisaruk BR, Watkins LR, Mayer DJ. Evidence for the neuropeptide cholecystokinin as an antagonist of opiate analgesia. *Science* 1983; 219: 310-312. Copyright 1983, AAAS.)

blocked by MK-329 (a CCK A receptor antagonist) and not by the CCK B antagonist L365,260. In contrast, the CCK B agonist BC264 produces a hyperalgesic effect that is antagonized by L365,260.[5] Similarly, when BDNL (a mixed CCK A & B agonist) is administered intracerebroventricularly, there is an antinociceptive response on both paw-lick and rat-jump responses. When BC264 (a selective CCK B agonist) is administered to the same location, a hyperalgesic response is detected. BDNL also potentiates the antinociceptive effects of the enkephalin-degrading enzyme inhibitor RB101 and the mu opioid agonist DAMGO, while BC264 reduces this effect.[6] As we have seen, endogenous CCK release occurs after opioid administration and after neural injury. To an extent, therefore, CCK seems to have a modulatory effect on opioid-derived analgesia.

The site of CCK release may also influence its effect. Injection of morphine into the rostro ventralmedial medulla (RVM) of the rat has been shown to attenuate the visceromotor effect of noxious colorectal distension in the rat, as measured electromyographically. This response is dose dependent. When CCK-8 is injected into the RVM, the visceromotor response to noxious colonic distension is enhanced. Conversely, administration of a selective CCK B, but not CCK A receptor antagonist significantly enhanced the antinociceptive response to morphine.[7]

Similar results were obtained by Kovelowski and colleagues (2000). Bilateral injection of lignocaine into the RVM was shown to block tactile allodynia and thermal hyperalgesia in spinal-nerve-ligated rats, but not sham-operated rats, in the absence of severe motor disturbance.[8] When L365,260 (a CCK B antagonist) is injected bilaterally into the RVM, a similar reduction in tactile allodynia and thermal hyperalgesia occurs. Injection of CCK-8 into the RVM of naïve rats produces a robust tactile allodynia effect and a more modest hyperalgesia, whereas morphine administration into the periaqueductal gray was significantly reduced in spinal-nerve-ligated rats. The injection of L365,260 into the RVM restored the potency of periaqueductal morphine in these spinal-nerve-ligated rats.[9] These results suggest that abnormal tonic activity in the descending facilitatory mechanisms may at least contribute to the chronic pain that arises from peripheral nerve injury. CCK and its interaction with opioids and their receptors seem important in this process. Heinricher and McGaraughty (1996) have reported that infusion of CCK-8 into the RVM attenuates the opioid-induced depression of ON cell activity in the RVM.[10] ON cells are thought to have a facilitatory influence on nociceptive processing through both local interactions within the RVM and descending systems projecting to the spinal cord as opposed to OFF cells, which are thought to comprise a descending inhibitory system that attenuates nociceptive information directly at the level of the spinal cord.[11-13]

Conversely, Jurna and Zetler (1981) found that a single injection of CCK-8 into the periaqueductal gray, caudate nucleus, and ventromedial thalamus produced a long-lasting inhibition of the tail-flick response to thermal stimulation. They also observed that when CCK-8 was administered in this fashion, sedation was observed. Naloxone abolished the antinociceptive, but not the sedative effects.[14]

Although the evidence presented here is not universally in keeping with an antiopioid effect of CCK, it does emphasize that CCK and the opioidergic systems are closely allied to and intrinsically involved with the actions of each other. The majority of the evidence suggests that CCK does reduce the analgesic effect of morphine, and hence by implication, other opioids. This effect is dependent on the type of CCK, be it the sulphated or nonsulphated, A or B varieties, the site to which the exogenous CCK is administered, and the dose that is applied.

The effect of exogenously administered CCK is only one part of, and a relatively small component of the overall evidence that CCK opposes the antinociceptive effect of opioids. The greater proportion of this evidence is contained in those studies which examine the effects of the specific CCK antagonists and their effects on opioid derived antinociception. This will be examined in subsequent chapters.

Chapter 9

Cholecystokinin Receptor Antagonists

A number of CCK antagonists have been synthesized and differ in their selectivity for the CCK A and B receptors, their absolute affinity, and their chemical structures. Since our emphasis is on CCK and its antagonists in relation to pain, the classification that relates to their selectivity for either receptor will be used.

Although many CCK receptor antagonists have been produced, our emphasis will be on those that are more usually described in the pain literature. Unlike CCK itself, CCK antagonists tend to be non-peptides and are hence amenable to oral administration as well as other forms of systemic application. When the literature is considered, confusion is possible. A variety of names are used for specific agents. For example, MK329 is the same as L364,718, which is also known as devazepide and which has been investigated in human practice under the trade name of Devakade.

A guide to the selectivity of various CCK antagonists is given in Table 9.1 while their affinities for the receptors are highlighted by Table 9.2.

MIXED CCK A AND B ANTAGONISTS

Proglumide

Proglumide is (Figure 9.1) a crystalline substance with a melting point of 142-145 °C. The LD_{50} in mice is 211-2,649 mg·kg^{-1} after IV administration, 7,350-8,861 mg·Kg^{-1} after oral use. It was originally patented in 1966.

Cholecystokinin and Its Antagonists in Pain Management
© 2006 by The Haworth Press, Inc. All rights reserved.
doi:10.1300/5593_09

TABLE 9.1. CCK receptor antagonists.

CCK A antagonists	CCK B antagonists	Mixed CCK A and B antagonists
T0632	L365,260	Proglumide
Asperlicin	(Colykade)	
MK 329/L364,718	L740,093	
(Devazepide)		
Loxiglumide	YM022	
Lorglumide	CI988	
PD135,666	PD135,158	
	L365,031	
	LY262,691	
	C2194	
	RP73870	
	YF476	

TABLE 9.2. Affinity data for CCK and CCK B antagonists.

CCK antagonist	CCK A affinity (nm)	CCK B affinity
Asperlicin[a]	1,400	$>10^5$
CI988[b]	2,717	1.7
Devazepide[c]	0.08	250
L365,260[c]	280	2
L365,031[d]	4.0	5,000
Lorglumide[e]	130	3.0×10^5
Loxiglumide[f]	330	9,100
LY262,691[g]	11,600	31
PD135,158[b]	1,232	2.8
PD135,666	40	0.2
Proglumide[e]	6.3×10^6	1.0×10^7
YM022[h]	316	0.05
L740,093[i]	>1,000	0.49

Sources: [a]Chang RS, Lotti VJ, Monaghan RL, Birnbaum J, Stapley E, Goetz M, Albers-Schonberg G, Patchett A, Liesch J. A potent nonpeptide cholecystokinin antagonist selective for peripheral tissues isolated from *Aspegillus alliaceus. Science* 1985; 230: 177-179; [b]Hughes J, Boden P, Costall B, Domeney A, Kelly E, Horwell D, Hunter J, Pinnock R, Woodruff G. Development of a class of selective cholecystokinin type B receptor antagonists having anxiolytic properties. *Proc Natl Acad Sci USA* 1990; 87: 6728-6732; [c]Lotti VJ, Chang RS. A new potent and selective non-peptide gastrin antagonist and brain cholecystokinin receptor (CCK-B) ligand: L365,260. *Eur J Pharmacol* 1989; 162: 273-280; [d]Hill DR, Campbell NJ, Shaw TM, Woodruff GN. Autoradiographic localization and biochemical characterization of peripheral type CCK receptors in rat CNS using highly selective nonpeptide CCK antagonists. *J Neurosci* 1987; 7: 2967-2976; [e]Makovec F, Bani M, Chiste R, Revel L, Rovati LC, Rovati LA. Differentiation of central and peripheral cholecystokinin receptors by new glutaramic acid derivatives with cholecystokinin-antagonistic activity. *Arzneim-Forsch Drug Res* 1986; 36: 98-102; [f]Freidinger RM. Cholecystokinin and gastrin antagonists. *Med Res Rev* 1989; 9: 271-290; [g]Howbert JJ, Lobb KL, Brown RF, Britton TC, Mason N. A novel series of non-peptide CCK and gastrin antagonists: Medicinal chemistry and electrophysiological demonstration of antagonism. In CT Dourish, SJ Cooper (Eds.), *Multiple cholecystokinin receptors: Progress towards CNS therapeutic targets* (pp. 28-37). London: Oxford University Press, London; [h]Dunlop J, Brammer N, Evans M, Ennis C. YM022 ((R)-1-[2,3-dihydro-1-(2'-methylphenacyl)-2-oxo-5-phenyl-1H-1,4-benzodiazepin-3-yl]-3-(3-methylphenyl)urea): An irreversible cholecystokinin type-B receptor antagonist. *Biochem Pharmac* 1997; 54: 81-85; [i]Dunlop J, Pass I, Ennis C. The cholecystokinin-B receptor antagonist L740,093 produces an insurmountable antagonism of CCK-4 stimulated functional responses in cells expressing the human CCK-B receptor. *Neuropeptides* 1998; 32: 157-160.

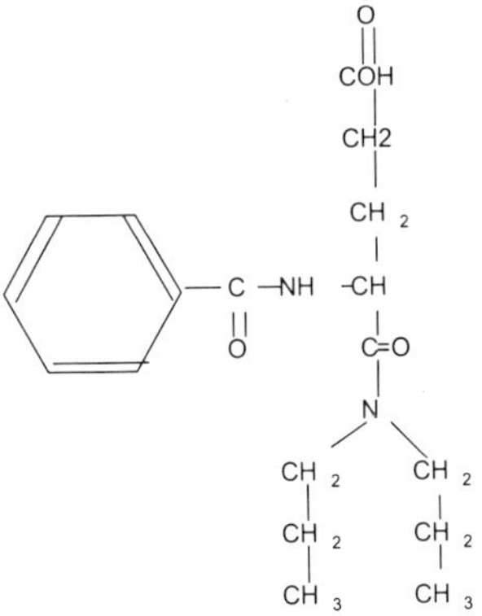

FIGURE 9.1. Proglumide (DL-4-benzamido-N,N-dipropylglutaramic acid).

Proglumide was originally used for its gastric effects. In a double-blind study comparing treatment with proglumide 1,200 mg day^{-1} and the H_2 antagonist cimetidine at a dose of 1,200 mg/day in patients with peptic ulcers, Galeone and colleagues (1978) showed that both drugs reduced both symptoms of peptic ulceration and gastric secretion in an equal fashion.[1] In another study examining the effect of proglumide on gastric ulcers, Miederer and colleagues (1979) compared in a double-blind fashion the effect of proglumide 1,200 mg/day with magnesium trisilicate. They found that the extent of ulcer healing as assessed by endoscopic examination was significantly greater and time to ulcer healing less in the proglumide group as opposed to the magnesium trisilicate group.[2] This ulcer healing effect is mediated by proglumide's CCK antagonistic properties,[3] which are of the mixed A and B variety. Bignamini and colleagues (1979) have suggested from their work in animal models that the terminal half-life of proglumide is about 24 hours.[4]

In adition to its effect on CCK receptors, proglumide may have intrinsic delta opioid effects. Rezvani and colleagues (1987) examined the effect of proglumide on isolated guinea pig ileum and the rat, mouse, and rabbit vas deferens. They found that proglumide inhibited the electrically stimulated twitches in the mouse vas deferens and guinea pig ileum but not in the rat or rabbit vas deferens. The inhibitory action of proglumide on the mouse vas deferens, but not guinea pig ileum, was antagonized by naloxone and by the selective delta-agonist ICI174,864 in a competitive fashion. They went on to study the in vitro binding of proglumide and found that proglumide displaces D-ala-D-[leucine][5]-enkephalin, a delta agonist, but not ethylketocyclazocine, a preferential kappa agonist. These results suggested that proglumide exerted opioid-like effects by activation of delta-opioid receptors.[5]

CCK A ANTAGONISTS

Asperlicin

Asperlicin, a nonpeptide CCK antagonist (Figure 9.2), was first isolated from the fungus *Aspergillus alliaceus*.[6] It has an affinity for CCK A receptors of about 300 to 400 times that of proglumide.[7] In vivo, it seems to be synthesized by *A. alliaceus* from tryptophan, anthanilate, and leucine.[8] A number of analogues of asperlicin have CCK antagonistic properties.[9-11]

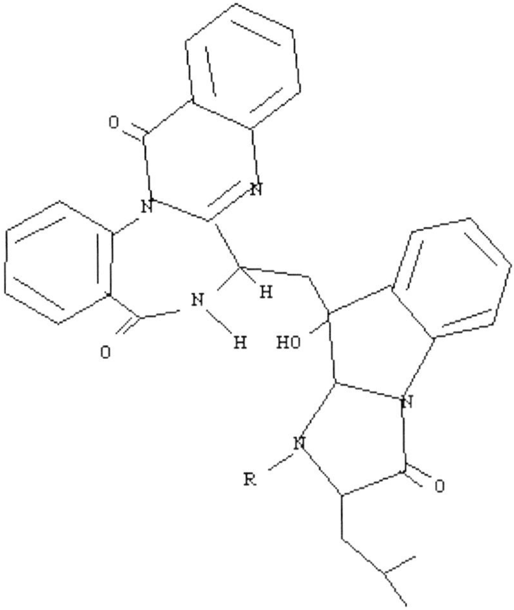

FIGURE 9.2. Asperlicin.

MK329/L364,718

Devazepide

Devazepide is a highly potent, nonpeptide, CCK A antagonist[12,13] that binds saturably and reversibly to CCK A receptors.[14] Its binding is stereospecific in that the more biologically active (-) enantiomer demonstrates more potency than the (+) enantiomer (see Figure 9.3).[14]

T0632

TO632, or sodium(S)-3-[1-(2-flurophenyl)-2,3-dihydro-3-[(3-iso-quinolinyl)-carbonyl]amino-6-methoxy-2-oxo-1-H-indole]propano-ate is a specific, reversible, highly potent CCK A antagonist[15] (See Figure 9.4).

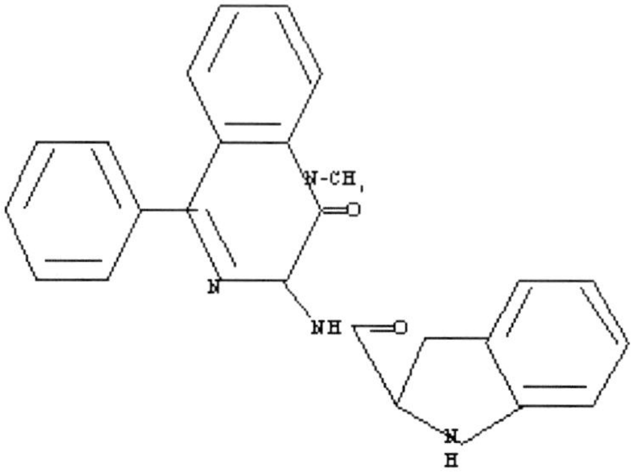

FIGURE 9.3. MK329/L364,718 (3S(-)-N-(2,3-dihydro-1-methyl-2-oxo-5-phenyl-1H-1,4-benzodiazepineyl)1H-indole-2-carboxamide) (*Source:* From Chang RS, Lotti VJ. Biochemical and pharmacological characterization of an extremely potent and selective nonpeptide cholecystokinin antagonist. *Proc Natl Acad Sci USA* 1986; 83: 4923-4926.)

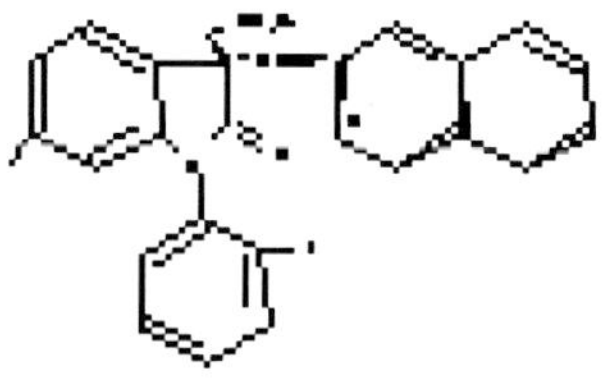

FIGURE 9.4. T0632 (sodium(S)-3-[1-(2-flurophenyl)-2,3-dihydro-3-[(3-iso-quinolinyl)-carbonyl]amino-6-methoxy-2-oxo-1-H-indole]propanoate).

Loxiglumide

CR1505

This glutaramic acid derivative (+/-)-4-(3,4-dicholrobenzamido)-N-(3-methoxypropyl)-N-pentylglutaramic acid is a selective CCK A antagonist.[16,17] Steady state is reached at approximately 48 hours after commencement of loxiglumide. Loxiglumide and its three main metabolites are excreted in the urine[18]. The absolute bioavailability after loxiglumide has been calculated is approximately 0.967[19] (see Figure 9.5).

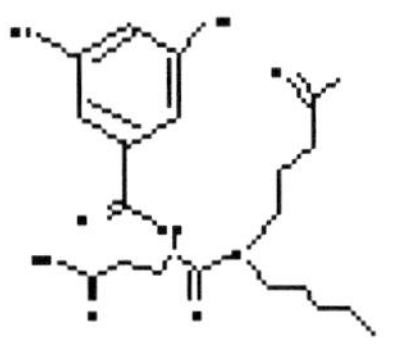

FIGURE 9.5. Loxiglumide.

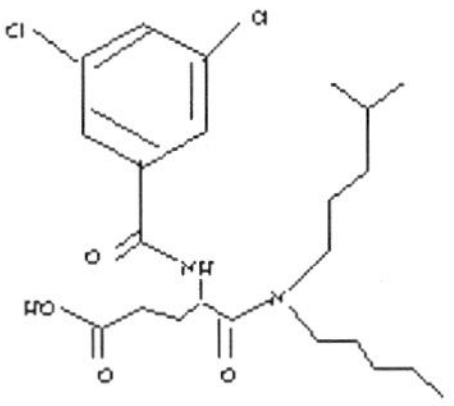

FIGURE 9.6. Lorglumide.

Lorglumide

CR1409

This potent, specific CCK A antagonist D,L-4-(3,4-dichloroben-zoylamino)-5-(dipentylamino)-5-oxo-pentanoic acid[20] which is about 4,000 times more potent in terms of its CCK receptor antagonism than proglumide[21] (see Figure 9.6).

CCK B ANTAGONISTS

L365,260

Colykade

Colykade is a white to off-white crystalline powder with a melting point of between 166.5 and 167.5 °C. The R enantiomer is approximately 100 times more potent than its S enantiomer in displacing binding at CCK B receptors.[22] Its affinity for CCK B receptors is around two magnitudes higher than its affinity for CCK A receptors.[22] After oral administration to rats, 98.5 percent is excreted in the feces within 96 hours. Biliary excretion is similarly high with 96 percent recovery from bile after 26 hours. In dogs, a higher percentage of L365,260 is found in urine. In vitro, L365,260 is highly protein bound (97.4 percent). Plasma half-life is around 100 minutes after oral administration in dogs, monkeys, and rats. LD_{50} in mice and rats is around 5,000 mg·Kg^{-1} after oral dose whereas figures of 2,500 mg·Kg^{-1} after intraperitoneal dosing in mice has been reported[23] (see Figure 9.7).

YM022

YM022, or [(R)-1-[2,3-dihydro-1-(2'methylphenacyl)-2-oxox-5-phenyl-1H-1,4-benzodiazepin-3-ly]-3-(3-methylphenyl)urea],[24] is a benzodiazepine structure that interacts with the CCK B receptor in an irreversible fashion.[24,25] Administration of YM022 significantly inhibits gastric acid secretion.[26,27] It exhibits a bell-shaped dose-response curve.[28] (see Figure 9.8).

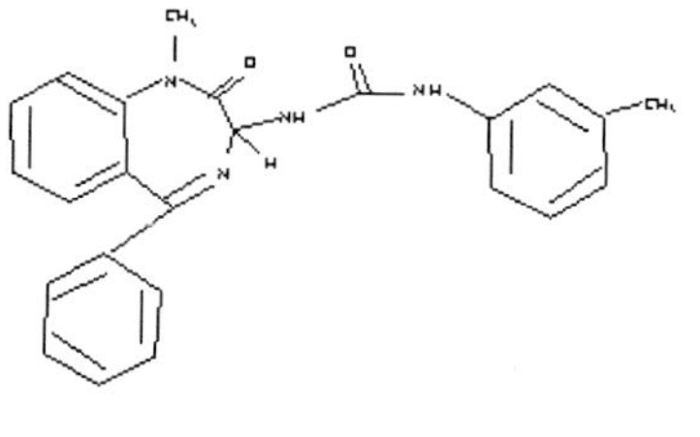

FIGURE 9.7. Colykade.

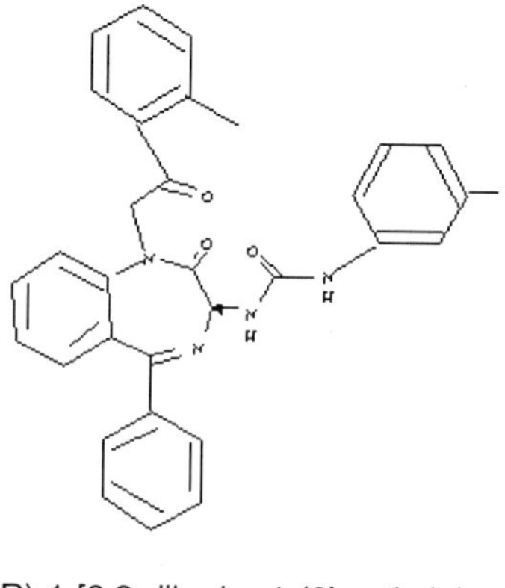

FIGURE 9.8. YM022 [(R)-1-[2,3-dihydro-1-(2'methylphenacyl)-2-oxox-5-phenyl-1H-1,4-benzodiazepin-3-ly]-3-(3-methylphenyl)urea].

YF476

YF476, or (3R)-N—(tert-butylcarbonylmethyl)-2,3-dihydro-2-oxo-5-(2-pyridyl-1,4-benzodiazepin-3-yl)-N'-(3-(methylamino)phenyl)urea, is an orally active CCK B antagonist with high oral bioavailability with an ED50 of 21 nmol·kg^{-1} in dogs.[29] (See Figure 9.9.)

ALTERNATIVE CLASSIFICATION

Normally, CCK antagonists are classified according to their relative affinities for either the CCK A or B receptors. An alternative classification is based on their chemical structures (see Table 9.3).

CCK ANTAGONISTS WITH OTHER EFFECTS

In addition to compounds with CCK antagonistic properties only, agents exist that are CCK antagonists and have other actions. As we will see later, CCK antagonists have a proanalgesic effect when used with opioids. The attraction of having a single therapeutic entity that combines this CCK and opioid effect is obvious. A variety of compounds have been investigated and been shown to possess this combined activity. One example, described by Hruby and colleagues (2003) is H-Tyr-DPhe-Gly-DTrp-NMeNle-Asp-Phe-NH$_2$ which combines CCK B antagonistic properties as well as potent delta and mu opioid agonistic activity.[30] Although this compound exemplifies what

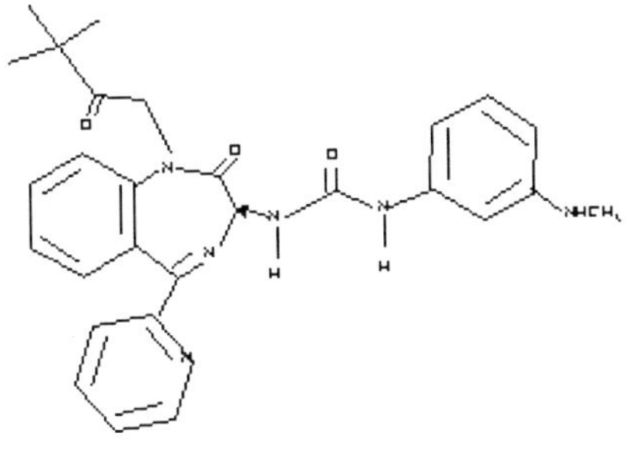

FIGURE 9.9. YF476 (3R)-N—(tert-butylcarbonylmethyl)-2,3-dihydro-2-oxo-5-(2-pyridyl-1,4-benzodiazepin-3-yl)-N'-(3-(methylamino)phenyl)urea.

TABLE 9.3. CCK antagonists according to chemical structure.

Peptoids	Nonpeptoids	1,4-benzodiazepines
Proglumide	Asperlicin	YM022
Lorglumide	MK329	L740,093
Loxiglumide	L365,260	YF476
CI988	LY262,691	
RP73870	T0632	

Source: Adapted from de Tullio P, Delarge J, Pirotte B. Recent advances in the chemistry of cholecystokinin receptor ligands (agonists and antagonists). *Curr Med Chem* 1999; 6: 433-455.

may be possible in terms of combining activity, its amino acid structure may mean that it is not suitable for oral administration.

A variety of agents are available that are antagonists at the CCK A, B, and both receptors. Individual agents differ in their affinity for these receptors and their pharmacokinetic profiles. Whether these differing affinities influence their ability to alter opioid-derived analgesia is still not clear. If antagonism at either receptor is associated with an alteration of opioid analgesia, then one might expect those agents with the greatest affinity for that receptor to have the greatest effect. In reality, this is not universally the case. The definite advantage of having specific CCK antagonists with high receptor affinity is that they can be used in experimental models to gain greater insight into the role of the CCK/opioidergic systems in nociceptive processing and to define the type of CCK, be it A or B, that is most important in that animal species with that particular type of pain.

The attraction of combining a CCK antagonist with an opioid agonist will become clearer in the next chapter where the effect of coadministration of a CCK antagonist with an opioid in experimental animals will be considered.

Chapter 10

Do Cholecystokinin Antagonists Influence Opioid-Derived Antinociception?

Although the effects of endogenous cholecystokinin on the gut and central nervous system are interesting, the real importance of CCK, and more particularly its antagonists, is the possibility of using these antagonists as therapeutic tools in pain treatment. Few would claim that even the strongest of opioids provide ideal pain relief for all sufferers. Dose escalation can increase effect, but may also increase side effects. If coadministration of another agent would enhance the analgesic effect of the opioid in question and allow either more complete pain relief, or the same level of pain relief using a lower dose of opioid, then the benefit would be obvious. CCK antagonists may represent one such therapeutic maneuver. In this chapter, we will examine some of the evidence derived from animal experimentation that examines the effect of a variety of CCK antagonists on opioid-derived nociception.

PROGLUMIDE

In 1985, Watkins and colleagues published the results of their work examining the effect of systemic administration of proglumide and morphine in rats. These drugs were given intraperitoneally, by the intrathecal route and also intracerebrally (into the periaqueductal gray matter). When proglumide, a mixed CCK A and B receptor antagonist, was administered alone, regardless of the route of administration, no antinociceptive effect, as assessed using a thermal tail-flick test, was observed. When morphine was given alone, an antinociceptive effect was observed, as would be expected. However, when proglumide and morphine were coadministered, the antinociceptive effect was enhanced.[1]

Bodnar and colleagues (1990) confirm these findings. They again used tail-flick latencies as their nociceptive test, but their experiments used mice. Proglumide again had no effect on flick latencies. Similarly, it did increase the antinociceptive effect of morphine in both animals that were tolerant to the antinociceptive effects of morphine and in morphine-naïve animals. This potentiation was proglumide-dose dependent. Proglumide shifted the dose response curve for morphine antinociception to the left and increased the duration of action of the morphine. They went on to show that subcutaneous proglumide enhanced the antinociceptive effect of intracerebroventricular [D-Ala^2, MePhe^4,Gly(ol)^5]enkephalin (DAGO) a highly selective mu$_1$ agonist but not [D-pen^2,D-Pen^5]enkephalin (DPDPE) a selective delta agonist. The selective mu$_1$ antagonist naloxonazine blocked proglumide-enhanced morphine analgesia.[2]

Zarrindast and colleagues (2000) provide a different perspective on the effect of proglumide. They studied mice on which spinal-nerve ligation was performed. Lick latencies were assessed and the effect of interventions on these lick latencies were used as a measure of the nociceptive or antinociceptive effect of that intervention. They found that when caerulein, a CCK agonist, was injected intracerebroventricularly, an antinociceptive effect was observed in the non-ligated, but not ligated animals. Morphine produced an antinociceptive effect in both ligated and nonligated mice, although the effect was less pronounced in ligated animals. A combination of caerulein and morphine produced an enhanced antinociceptive effect, which was more prominent in ligated animals. As with the studies previously mentioned, proglumide alone had no antinociceptive effect in active or control animals, but enhanced the antinociceptive effect of caerulein in ligated animals.[3]

PD134,308/CI988

In contrast to the lack of antinociceptive effect of proglumide when administered alone, Wiesenfeld-Hallin and colleagues (1990) found that in rats, the selective CCK B antagonist PD134,308 produced a weak and naloxone-reversible depression of the flexor reflex and antinociceptive effect in the hot plate test. This effect was significantly greater when morphine was coadministered. The response to PD134,308 was dose related and even when 30-fold greater doses of PD134,308 were given, there was no evidence of the bell-shaped dose response curve apparent when L365,260 is used[4] (Figure 10.1).

Coudore-Civiale and colleagues studied the effects of CI988 (also known as PD134,308) in normal, mono-neuropathic, and diabetic rats. CI988 had no antinociceptive effects in normal rats but had a definite antinociceptive effect in the mono-neuropathic and diabetic rats. When CI988 was used in combination with morphine, there was a superadditive effect in terms of antinociception in the diabetic rats only. Indeed, an ineffective dose of CI988, when combined with an ineffective dose of morphine produced a definite antinociceptive effect. CI988 also had an anti-allodynic effect, albeit weak, in the mono-neuropathic, but not diabetic rats.[5] Others have shown that

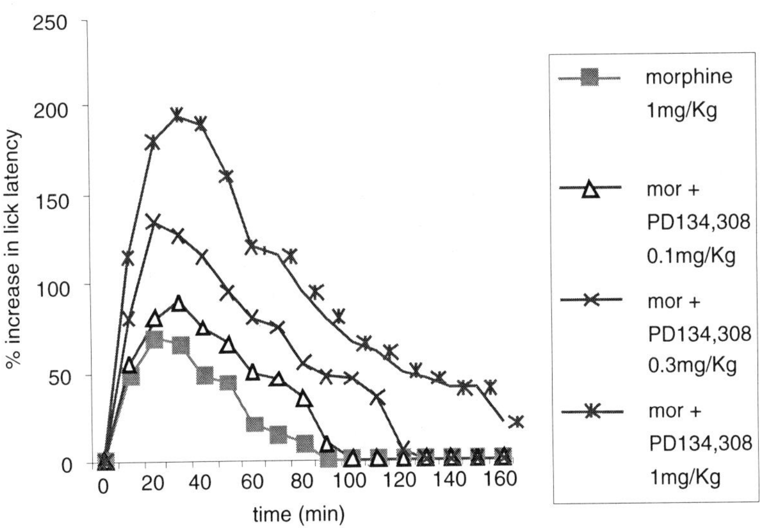

FIGURE 10.1. Effect of 1 mg·Kgn[-1] morphine by itself and in combination with PD134,308 at various doses. (*Source:* Wiesenfeld-Hallin Z, Xu X-J, Hughes J, Horwell DC, Hokfelt T. PD134,308, a selective antagonist of cholecystokinin type B receptor, enhances the analgesic effect of morphine and synergistically interacts with galanin to depress spinal nociceptive reflexes. *Proc Natl Acad Sci USA* 1990; 87: 7105-7109. Reprinted with permission.)

CI988 has a significant antinociceptive effect after peripheral nerve injury.[6]

L365,260

In one of the few studies performed in primates, O'Neill and colleagues (1990) studied the antinociceptive effects in squirrel monkeys using a monkey tail withdrawal to a thermal stimulus. L365,260, a CCK B antagonist, significantly elevated withdrawal latencies suggesting an antinociceptive effect produced by L365,260.[7]

A more complicated insight into the effects of L365,260 is given by Nichols and colleagues (1995). This group studied nociception in nerve-ligated rats. Such animals displayed signs of allodynia. In the doses studied, morphine had no anti-allodynic effect. DAMGO [D-ALA^2,NMPhe^4,Gly-ol]enkephalin, a high-efficacy mu-opioid agonist, did produce a dose-dependent anti-allodynic effect. In contrast, the delta opioid agonist [D-Ala^2,Glu^4]deltorphin was anti-allodynic only at the highest doses studied, and this effect was not total. When morphine and [D-Ala^2,Glu^4]deltorphin were administered together at doses in which neither was anti-allodynic alone, significant and long-lasting reductions in allodynia were observed. This effect was antagonized by naltrindole (a delta antagonist). L365,260 had no effect when given alone, but did produce a significant anti-allodynic effect when given with morphine, an effect that was abolished if naltrindole was also given.[8] Again we see that an inactive dose of morphine can be rendered active by coadministration of a CCK antagonist.

PD135,158

Yamamoto and Sakashita (1999) studied the effects of morphine alone and in combination with PD135,158 in two rat models of neuropathic pain, the chronic constriction injury, and sciatic nerve injury models. Antinociception was measured by the paw-withdrawal latency to thermal nociceptive stimuli. All drugs were administered by the intrathecal route. In the chronic constriction injury model, intrathecal morphine increased the paw-withdrawal latencies of injured and uninjured paws. PD135,158 potentiated the antinociceptive effect of morphine on injured and uninjured paws. In the partial sciatic injury model, the effect of morphine on the injured paw was less potent than that on the uninjured paw and PD135,158 potentiated the morphine-induced antinociception in the uninjured, and had only a minor effect on the morphine analgesia in the injured paw.[9]

COMPARISONS BETWEEN CCK ANTAGONISTS

Comparing the effect of various CCK antagonists, each with known receptor affinity, may allow conclusions to be made regarding the relative importance of the individual receptors in relation to opioid-derived antinociception. Although this approach has much to commend it, the majority of animal studies have been performed in rodent and murine models and there is a danger in extrapolating these results to primate and human practice.

Proglumide versus L365,260 versus L364,718

Friederich and Gebhart (2000) examined the actions of morphine and three separate CCK antagonists in a rat visceral pain model. Colonic distension was used as a nociceptive stimulus and animals with colonic inflammation (induced by instillation of 2,4,6-trinitrobenzenesulfonic acid [TNBS]) and animals inflammation free were studied.

After repetitive TNBS instillation, visceromotor responses to colonic distension was increased. Morphine had a greater antinociceptive effect in those with colonic distension. The mixed CCK A and B antagonist proglumide, when administered intrathecally, dose dependently enhanced the antinociceptive effect of morphine in vehicle, but not TNBS-treated rats. Similarly, use of the CCK B antagonist was associated with a dose-dependent increase in the antinociceptive effects of morphine in those animals without colonic inflammation. In contrast, when L364,718, a specific CCK A antagonist was used, there was no enhancement of the antinociceptive effect of morphine in animals with or without colonic inflammation.[10] These results suggest that the CCK B receptor is important in the modulation of morphine-derived antinociception, at least in the rat. When inflammation of the colon is present, this enhancing effect of CCK B antagonists is lost.

L364,718 versus L365,260

Lavigne and colleagues (1992) again used a rat thermal sensorimotor tail-flick test when assessing the antinociceptive effects of morphine used alone and in combination with CCK antagonists. They found that both L364,718 (a CCK A antagonist) and L365,260 (a CCK B antagonist) significantly enhanced the antinociceptive effect of morphine, but only in rats that had not been acclimated to the laboratory environment or habituated to handling by the investigators.[11] This enhancement of morphine antinociception by both L365, 260 and L364,718 reported by Lavigne and colleagues (1992) is consistent with the results of Dourish and colleagues (1988 and 1990) who demonstrated a similar effect with similar doses of morphine.[12,13] Lavigne's and colleagues' results suggest that the pharmacological response to morphine and CCK antagonists may be modified by factors related to the behavioral state of the experimental animal. This suggestion is consistent with the observation that results from nociceptive testing in animals is influenced by the duration and frequency of restraint,[14] exposure to a predator,[15] and to attentional influences.[16]

Lorglumide versus PD135,158

When lorglumide or PD135,158 is injected alone, intracerebroventricularly in the mouse, no change from baseline tail-flick response is observed. Injection of CCK-8 antagonizes the antinociceptive effect of morphine, beta-endorphin, and kappa opioid agonist USO, 488H except when PD135,158 is coadministered. The intracerebroventricular administration of lorglumide dose-dependently blocks the antagonistic effect of CCK-8 on beta-endorphin and U50,488H-induced, but not morphine-induced inhibition of the tail-flick response suggesting that both CCK A and B receptors are involved in antagonizing the antinociceptive effect of beta-endorphin and U50,488H, but only the B receptor antagonizes the effect of morphine.[17]

PD140,548 versus CI988

Singh and colleagues (1996) examined the effect of these CCK antagonists on morphine-induced antinociception. Neither CI988 (a

CCK B antagonist) nor PD140,548 (a CCK A antagonist) possessed any antinociceptive effect in any of their nociceptive tests. CI988 was associated, at least at the lower dose levels, with a potentiation of morphine-induced antinociception as assessed with a radiant heat model of the tail flick-test, the acute phase of the formalin test, and during the tonic phase of the same test. CI988 was ineffective in potentiating morphine antinociception at higher dose levels. In contrast, PD140,548 was associated with a potentiation of morphine antinociception only during the tonic phase of the formalin test.[18] This bell-shaped dose-response curve with CI988 is similar to that found with L365,360.[13]

FK480 versus YM022

Yamamoto and Nozaki-Taguchi (1996) studied the effects of these CCK antagonists on the pain caused by paw formalin injection in rats. Typically, formalin injection produces a two-phase response: a short, phase one followed by a longer, phase two response. Any antinociceptive effect can be assessed by measuring the flinching response to the formalin injection. When the CCK A antagonist FK480 is given intrathecally either before or after formalin injection, no alteration in the normal response was observed. In contrast, when YM022 is given intrathecally prior to formalin injection, there is a dose-dependent reduction in flinching behavior.

Treatment with YM022 after formalin injection failed to alter the normal response. The antinociceptive effect of pretreatment with YM022 was unaltered by naloxone, suggesting that the response was not mediated by spinal opioid-receptor activation[19] (Figure 10.2). The mechanisms underlying the depression of formalin-induced flinching behavior after CCK B blockade is not known. CCK B receptor activation increases basal release of endogenous excitatory amino acids, such as glutamate and aspartate in rat hippocampal slices and CCK B antagonists completely reverse this process.[20]

Proglumide versus Lorglumide

Although the evidence presented up until now has suggested that CCK antagonists enhance morphine-induced antinociception, the work of Kellstein and Mayer (1990) introduces a potentially negative

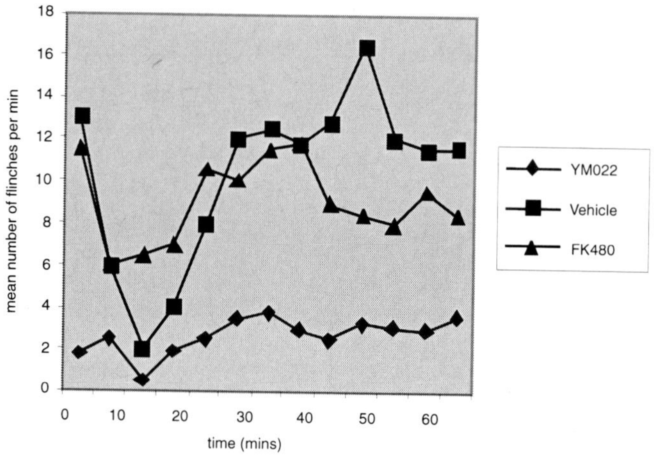

FIGURE 10.2. Number or flinches after formalin injection: Pretreatment with intrathecal YM022, FK480, and vehicle. (*Source:* Reproduced with permission from Yamamoto T, Nozaki-Taguchi N. The effects of intrathecally administered FK480, a cholecystokinin-A receptor antagonist, and YM022, a cholecystokinin-B receptor antagonist, on the formalin test in the rat. *Anesth Analg* 1996; 83: 107-113.)

aspect. They found that while lorglumide (a CCK A antagonist) and proglumide (a mixed CCK A and B antagonist) had no antinociceptive effect (as measured with a rat tail-flick test) when given alone, both significantly increased morphine antinociception when given with that analgesic. However, this effect was only apparent for the first week after initiation of daily treatment. From days 8 to 15 neither proglumide nor lorglumide had any effect on the antinociceptive effect of the morphine. After day 15, repeated administration of either CCK antagonist with morphine was associated with an attenuation of its effect. When treatment with either CCK antagonist was discontinued, within a short period of time, a return to the original situation of enhancement of morphine antinociception with either CCK antagonist was apparent. They further noted that there was a bell-shaped dose-response curve with both proglumide and lorglumide.[21] Although they were unable to offer a conclusive reason for this loss of morphine enhancement with chronic use of these CCK antagonists, they did suggest that there may have been an up-regulation of CCK receptors to account for the finding. Neither proglumide nor lorglumide have a high affinity for the CCK B receptor and the majority of work undertaken in rodent models suggests that the most significant enhancement of morphine antinociception is associated with antagonism of the CCK B receptor.

CCK ANTAGONISTS AND ENKEPHALINS

Although evidence supports the contention that administration of a CCK antagonist with morphine can enhance the antinociceptive effect of morphine, this approach still relies on the administration of a strong opioid. The appeal of gaining an analgesic effect by administering a CCK antagonist alone to enhance the analgesic effect of endogenous enkephalins is appealing. If one could further augment the concentration of those enkephalins, then this too would be appealing. Evidence that both strategies may be possible exists.

CCK Antagonists and Endogenous Enkephalins

Extracellular levels of enkephalins can be raised by the enkephalin-degrading enzyme inhibitor RB101[22] and such elevation is associated with dose-dependent antinociception, which is naloxone-reversible.[23] Valverde and colleagues (1994) studied the effect of three CCK B antagonists, L365,260, PD134,308, and RB211 on enkephalin-mediated antinociception using a rat tail-flick and mouse hot-plate tests. All three CCK B antagonists strongly potentiated the antinociceptive effects of RB101 in the rat tail-flick test. Indeed, the antinociception observed after coadministration of RB101 and L365, 260, RB211, and PD134,308 was 300, 500, and 800 percent higher, respectively, than that observed when RB101 was given alone. This effect was partially blocked by naloxone. In the mouse hot-plate test, all three CCK B antagonists again increased the extent of antinociception produced by RB101, but in this case by about two times less than in the case of the rat tail-flick test.[24]

Valverde and colleagues examined the effect of RB101 when used in conjunction with CI988 (a CCK B antagonist) in a rat diabetic neuropathic pain model. When RB101 was used alone there was a suppression of mechanical hyperalgesia (paw pressure vocalization threshold), and a partial alleviation of mechanical allodynia (von Frey hair test), but it was ineffective for thermal allodynia. Its effects were blocked by naloxone and naltrindole (mu and delta antagonists). The combination of an inactive dose of CI988 and the lowest effective dose of RB101 resulted in a greater increase in vocalization threshold than when RB101 was used alone.[25]

Another potential application for enkephalinase inhibitors and CCK antagonists is use during morphine withdrawal. When PD134, 308 is given alone, no decrease in the signs of naloxone-precipitated morphine withdrawal is observed. RB101 does significantly decrease these signs when given alone, but this effect is enhanced when it is given in combination with PD134,308.[26] Maldonado and colleagues (1995) who defined this effect, also investigated the potential mechanism of this effect. They found that both PD134,308 and RB101 inhibited the binding of [3H]-diprenorphine binding to opioid receptors in mice[26] suggesting that both agents produce an increase in enkephalin levels.

Perhaps the major drawback associated with the use of RB101 is its relatively short half-life. Enkephalins are inactivated by two metallopeptidases, neutral endopeptidase and aminopeptidase N, which can be blocked by dual inhibitors. One such inhibitor is RB3007, a systemically active prodrug, which has a longer duration of action than RB101. When RB3007 is administered to mice, long-lasting antinociceptive effects, as observed in the hot-plate test, are observed. These effects are blocked by naloxone. Similar effects were observed in the rat tail-flick test, writhing and formalin tests in mice, and the paw-pressure test in the rat. Injection of RB3007 significantly increased the extracellular levels of Met-enkephalin and this increase mirrors the antinociceptive effects observed. The CCK B antagonist PD134,308 and the opioid agonist methadone, when given in subanalgesic doses, significantly increased the antinociception observed with RB3007 use.[27]

Vanderah and colleagues (1995) examined the effect of L365,260 in mice. Intracerebroventricular (i.c.v.) L365,260 did not produce any antinociceptive effects in the mouse warm-water tail-flick test. Similarly, i.c.v. thiorphan, a peptidase inhibitor, did not produce any antinociceptive effect. However, when both L365,260 and thiorphan were given together, a significant antinociceptive effect was observed. This effect was blocked by naltrindole (a delta antagonist) or antisera to [Leu[5]]enkephalin, but not antisera to [Met[5]]enkephalin.[28] [Leu[5]]enkephalin seems to act as a ligand for the delta opioid receptor. These results suggest that the combination of endogenous opioids and this CCK B antagonist produce an effect mediated by delta-opioid receptors. This is supported by the finding that specific antisera to the delta-opioid receptor agonist [Leu[5]]enkephalin attenuates the antinociceptive effect produced by L365,260 and thiorphan. CCK may act to tonically inhibit the release, availability, or degradation of endogenous [Leu[5]]enkephalin or a similar substance.

CCK ANTAGONISTS AND TRICYCLIC ANTIDEPRESSANTS

Although the major focus of this chapter has been on the effect on antinociception produced by the combination of CCK antagonists and opioids, a fascinating glimpse at the possible complementary effect of CCK antagonists and tricyclic antidepressants (TCAs) is given by the work of Coudore-Civiale and colleagues (2000). They examined the effects of intrathecally administered CI988 (a CCK B antagonist) on the antinociceptive effects of intravenous morphine and clomipramine in diabetic rats. Antinociception was measured using a paw-pressure threshold test. As would be expected, both morphine and clomipramine, when given alone, had an antinociceptive effect. CI988, in keeping with the results of Wiesenfeld-Hallin and colleagues (1990),[4] also had a modest antinociceptive effect. However, when a combination of CI988 and clomipramine were used together, the antinociceptive effect produced was significantly greater than that produced by either agent when used alone[29] (Figure 10.3).

This interaction between a CCK antagonist and a TCA may be explained by a possible effect on serotonin produced by CCK antagonists.

Fluvoxamine, a serotonin blocking agent, induces a decrease in the sensitivity of panic disorder patients to CCK-4.[30] However, other studies have failed to show any interaction between CCK and the serotinergic system.[31] An alternative explanation revolves around the observation that at least some of the antinociceptive effects of the TCAs may involve opioidergic mechanisms and that their antinociceptive effects can be inhibited by naloxone.[32]

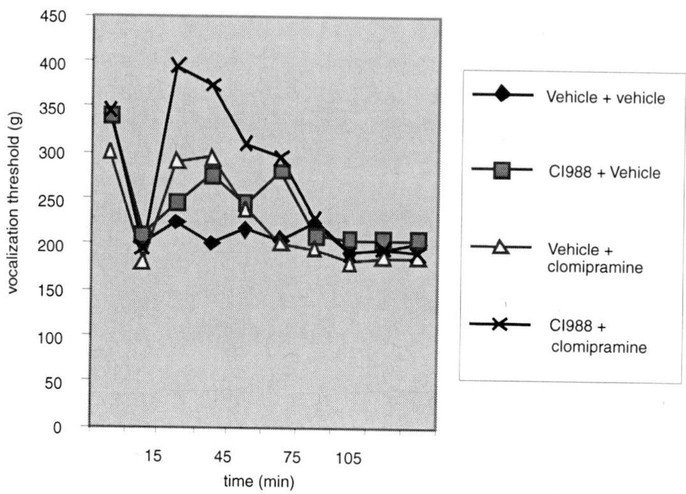

FIGURE 10.3. Effect of combination of intrathecal vehicle + intravenous vehicle, intrathecal CI988 + intravenous vehicle, intrathecal vehicle + intravenous clomipramine, and intrathecal CI988 + intravenous clomipramine on rat vocalization thresholds. (*Source:* Reprinted from *Neuroscience Letters,* 286, Coudore-Civiale MA, Courteix C, Boucher M, Meen M, Fialip J, Eschalier A, and Ardid D. Potentiation of morphine and clomipramine analgesia by cholecystokinin-B antagonist t CI988 in diabetic rats, pp. 37-40, copyright 2000, with permission from Elsevier.)

SUMMARY

Of the CCK antagonists, an antinociceptive effect is only associated with CI988 when it is used alone. The others require addition of either morphine or an enkephalinase inhibitor for an antinociceptive, or rather an enhancement of the antinociceptive effect of the coadministered agent, to be apparent. The majority of the work arising from animal experimentation suggests that the greatest enhancement of opioid-derived antinociception is produced when CCK B antagonists are used. This corresponds to the finding of a predominance of CCK B and its receptor in the central nervous system as compared to CCK A, which is more extensively represented in the gut, at least in the common animal models.

The other consistent finding from these experiments is that a subtherapeutic dose of CCK antagonist combined with a subtherapeutic dose of opioid can produce definite antinociception (see Table 10.1). The implications for human practice are obvious. The majority of the studies described were performed in murine or rodent models. Only one was performed in primates, namely the squirrel monkey. Therefore, the question arises as to whether it is legitimate to predict from these experiments the likely results in human clinical practice. Furthermore, is CCK B and its receptors predominant in the human CNS as in the rodent and murine models? Do CCK antagonists have a similar effect on opioid-derived pain relief in humans as demonstrated in the animal work and are the results obtained when CCK antagonists are used with morphine reproduced when other opioids such as codeine, fentanyl, tramadol, oxycodone, and meperidine are used? As we will see in later chapters, only some of the answers to these questions exist.

TABLE 10.1. Summary of evidence relating to potentiation of antinociceptive effects of morphine and enkephalinase inhibitors with CCK antagonists.

CCK antagonist	Type	Antinociceptive effect		
		Alone	With morphine	With enkephalinase inhibitor
Proglumide	A&B	no[a,b,c]	yes[a,b,d,e]	
CI988	B	yes[f,g,h] no[i]	yes[f,g,i]	yes[j,k,l]
L365,260	B	no[m,n]	yes[e,m,o,p,q,r]	yes[j,n]
PD135,158	B	no[c]	yes[s,t]	
YM022	B	yes[u]		
RB211	B			yes[j]
FK480	A	no[u]		
L364,718	A		yes[p,g,r] no[e]	
Lorglumide	A	no[c,t]	yes[t]	
PD140,548	A	no[i]	yes[i]	

Sources: [a]Bodnar RJ, Paul D, Pasternak GW. Proglumide selectively potentiates supraspinal mu_1 opioid analgesia in mice. *Neuropharmacology* 1990; 29:

507-510; [b]Zarrindast M-R, Samiee F, Rezayat M. Antinociceptive effect of intracerebroventricular administration of cholecystokinin receptor agonist and antagonist in nerve-ligated mice. *Pharmacol Toxicol* 2000; 87: 169-173; [c]Kellstein DE, Mayer DJ. Chronic administration of cholecystokinin antagonists reverses the enhancement of spinal morphine analgesia induced by acute pretreatment. *Brain Res* 1990; 516: 263-270; [d]Watkins LR, Kinscheck IB, Mayer DJ. Potentiation of morphine analgesia by the cholecystokinin antagonist proglumide. *Brain Res* 1985; 327: 169-180; [e]Friederich AE, Gebhart GF. Effects of spinal cholecystokinin receptor antagonists on morphine antinociception in a model of visceral pain in the rat. *J Pharmacol Exp Ther* 2000; 292: 538-544; [f]Wiesenfeld-Hallin Z, Xu X-J, Hughes J, Horwell DC, Hokfelt T. PD134,308, a selective antagonist of cholecystokinin type B receptor, enhances the analgesic effect of morphine and synergistically interacts with galanin to depress spinal nociceptive reflexes. *Proc Natl Acad Sci USA* 1990; 87: 7105-7109; [g]Coudore-Civiale M-A, Courteix C, Fialip J, Boucher M, Eschalier A. Spinal effect of the cholecystokinin-B receptor antagonist CI-988 on hyperalgesia, allodynia and morphine-induced analgesia in diabetic and mononeuropathic rats. *Pain* 2000; 88: 15-22; [h]Coudore-Civiale MA, Courteix C, Boucher M, Meen M, Fialip J, Eschalier A, and Ardid D. Potentiation of morphine and clomipramine analgesia by cholecystokinin-B antagonist CI988 in diabetic rats. *Neurosci Lett* 2000; 286: 37-40; [i]Singh L, Oles RJ, Field MJ, Atwal P, Woodruff GN, Hunter JC. Effect of CCK receptor antagonists on the antinociceptive, reinforcing and gut motility properties of morphine. *Br J Pharmacol* 1996; 118: 1317-1325; [j]Valverde O, Maldonado R, Fournie-Zaluski MC, Roques BP. Cholecystokinin B antagonists strongly potentiate antinociception mediated by endogenous enkephalins. *J Pharmacol Exp Ther* 1994; 270: 77-88; [k]Coudore-Civiale MA, Meen M, Fournie-Zaluski MC, Boucher M, Roques BP, Eschalier A. Enhancement of the effects of a complete inhibitor of enkephalin-catabolizing enzymes, RB101, by a cholecystokinin B receptor antagonist in diabetic rats. *Br J Pharmacol* 2001; 133: 179-185; [l]Le Guen S, Nieto MM, Canestrelli C, Chen H, Fournie-Zaluski MC, Cupo A, Maldonado R, Roques BP, and Noble F. Pain management by a new series of dual inhibitors of enkephalin degrading enzymes: Long lasting antinociceptive properties and potentiation by CCK_2 antagonist or methadone. *Pain* 2003; 104: 139-148; [m]Nichols ML, Bian D, Ossipov MH, Lai J, Porreca F. Regulation of morphine antiallodynia efficacy by cholecystokinin in a model of neuropathic pain in rats. *J Pharmacol Exp Ther* 1995; 275: 1339-1345; [n]Vanderah TW, Bernstein RN, Lai J, Porreca F. Production of naltrindole-sensitive antinociception by a cholecystokinin (CCK) antagonist and thiorphan: evidence for tonic inhibition of enkephalin release by CCK. *Analgesia* 1995; 1: 813-816; [o]O'Neill MF, Dourish CT, Tye SJ, Iversen SD. Blockade of CCK-B receptors by L365,260 induces analgesia in the squirrel monkey. *Brain Res* 1990; 534: 287-290; [p]Lavigne GJ, Millington WR, Mueller GP. The CCK-A and CCK-B receptor antagonists, Devazepide and L365,260, enhance morphine antinociception only in non-acclimated rats exposed to a novel environment. *Neuropeptides* 1992; 21: 119-129; [q]Dourish CT, Hawley D, Iversen SD. Enhancement of morphine analgesia and prevention of morphine tolerance in the rat by the cholecystokinin antagonist L364,718. *Eur J Pharmacol* 1988; 147: 469-472; [r]Dourish CT, O'Neill MF, Coughlan J, Kitchener SJ, Hawley D, Iversen SD. The selective CCK-B receptor antagonist L365,260 enhances morphine analgesia and prevents morphine tolerance in the rat. *Eur J Pharmacol* 1990; 176: 35-44; [s]Yamamoto T, Sakashita Y. Differential effects of intrathecally administered morphine and its interaction with cholecystokinin-B antagonist on thermal hyperalgesia following two models of experimental mononeuropathy in the rat. *Anesthesiology* 1999; 90: 1382-1391; [t]Suh HW, Kim Y-H, Choi YS, Song DK. Involvement of different subtypes of cholecystokinin receptors in opioid antinociception in the mouse. *Peptides* 1995; 16: 1229-1234; [u]Yamamoto T, Nozaki-Taguchi N. The effects of intrathecally administered FK480, a cholecystokinin-A receptor antagonist, and YM022, a cholecystokinin-B receptor antagonist, on the formalin test in the rat. *Anesth Analg* 1996; 83: 107-113.

Chapter 11

Do CCK Antagonists Reduce Tolerance to the Antinociceptive Effects of Opioids?

The current trend for increased use of strong opioids in human clinical practice is based on a firm body of evidence that this class of agents can be effective for a variety of pain conditions, including those which are of a chronic nature. Despite this trend, few would argue that they are universally effective as analgesics or devoid of side effects. In many cases, their analgesic effect and incidence of side effects associated with their use are dose related. In addition, their use may be complicated by analgesic tolerance, that is, a need to increase dose in order to achieve the same level of analgesia. At worst, the patient may take the strong opioid and be completely tolerant to its analgesic effect. Stopping the opioid may not be possible due to withdrawal effects. Although it is still not clear exactly how much of an issue analgesic tolerance is in human clinical practice with either weak or strong opioids, any intervention that could lessen this potential side effect would be helpful, more so if this intervention was not associated with the addition of extra side effects. A body of evidence suggests that one such therapeutic intervention could be the use of CCK antagonists. This evidence is entirely from the field of animal experimentation. As yet, no similar work has been undertaken in humans, but then again, no serious attempt has yet been made to define the nature and extent of analgesic tolerance with weak and strong opioids in human practice either.

Cholecystokinin and Its Antagonists in Pain Management

doi:10.1300/5593_11

EFFECT OF CCK ANTAGONISTS ON ANTINOCICEPTIVE EFFECT OF OPIODS

The notion that CCK antagonists may influence antinociceptive tolerance to the effects of opioids is not new. In 1984, Watkins and colleagues described the effect of proglumide when administered in a number of experimental situations. They confirmed the observation that the antinociceptive effect of morphine is enhanced by intrathecal proglumide at lower doses and an attenuation of antinociception at higher doses. Furthermore, enkephalin-mediated antinociception, as produced by front-paw footshock analgesia or by exogenous administration of the enkephalin analog [D-Ala^2]methionine enkephalinamide (DALA) was again potentiated by proglumide. They went on to examine the effect of proglumide on antinociceptive tolerance. Tolerance was produced by twice daily intraperitoneal injection of increasing doses of morphine. When antinociception was measured, there were no differences in the results between animals receiving a further dose of morphine or vehicle, indicating that tolerance had occurred. In contrast, when proglumide was administered to the tolerant rats and a further dose of morphine given, an antinociceptive effect was apparent.[1]

Tang and colleagues (1984) reported similar results. Again using a rat model, they found that acute tolerance to the antinociceptive effects of morphine could be produced by seven to eight subcutaneous injections of morphine. If proglumide was coadministered with the morphine, the tolerance produced was of a lesser magnitude. In those animals who received only morphine and who had become tolerant, antinociception to further doses of morphine was produced by the addition of proglumide, indicating that the proglumide had reversed the tolerance to morphine. They also sampled CSF in these rats and found that the continual administration of morphine increased CSF CCK levels.[2]

Panerai and colleagues (1987) again studied the effects of proglumide (and the CCK antagonist benzotript) on morphine tolerance. Rats were chronically treated with morphine, proglumide, or benzotript alone. Those animals treated with proglumide or benzotript derived no antinociceptive effect. Tolerance was assessed by administering graded doses of morphine and using the tail-flick and hot-plate tests. When proglumide or benzotript was given to the rats along with a dose of morphine after chronic oral morphine use, the morphine dose-response curve was displaced to the right when compared to animals treated with placebo suggesting that tolerance was reversed by use of a CCK antagonist.

EFFECT ON MORPHINE DEPENDENCE

They also examined the effect of these CCK antagonists on morphine dependance as judged by the reaction to acute naloxone administration. After chronic morphine administration, the effects of proglumide or benzotript treatment along with naloxone were no different to when naloxone was administered alone suggesting that these CCK antagonists had no effect on morphine dependence.[3]

This lack of effect of a CCK antagonist on the development of morphine dependence, as precipitated by naloxone injection after chronic morphine treatment is confirmed by Dourish and colleagues (1988). In their study, the CCK A antagonist L364,718 was used. They also confirm that this CCK antagonist can prevent the onset of morphine antinociceptive tolerance. Rats were treated with morphine, placebo, or morphine and L364,718. After six days, those animals treated with morphine alone displayed features of morphine tolerance, while those treated with an equal dose of morphine along with L364,718 were still getting close to baseline levels of antinociception from morphine administration.[4]

Dourish and colleagues also examined the effect of the CCK A antagonist L365,031 and the CCK B antagonist L365,260 on morphine-derived antinociception. Neither L365,031 nor L365,260 had any effect on baseline pain thresholds in the radiant heat tail-flick test or paw-pressure test. As would be expected, they both enhanced the antinociceptive effect of morphine when given acutely. As before, rats were given morphine twice daily and became tolerant to its antinociceptive effects. Twice daily injections of L365,031 or L365, 260 prevented the development of tolerance to the effects of morphine[5] (Figure 11.1).

Idanpaan-Heikkila and colleagues (1997) have shown that the prevention of tolerance with morphine is also observed in an experimental neuropathic pain model. Rats had a surgically induced unilateral peripheral neuropathy inflicted (Bennett and Xie model). At day 12

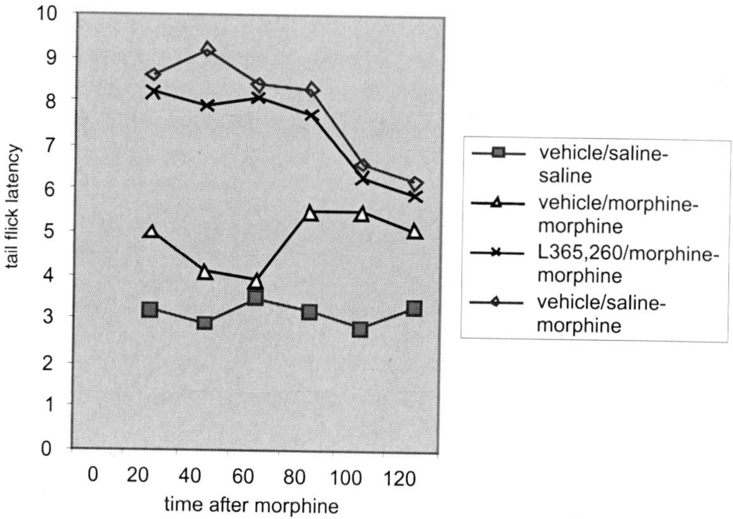

FIGURE 11.1. Prevention of tolerance to morphine analgesia by the CCK B antagonist L365,260 in the rat tail-flick test. Tolerance produced by twice daily morphine injection. Effect of morphine for six days then further dose of morphine, morphine with L365,260 then additional morphine, vehicle and saline then saline injection and vehicle and saline for 6 days followed by further saline. (*Source:* Reprinted from *Eur J Pharmacol,* 176, Dourish CT, O'Neill MF, Coughlan J, Kitchener SJ, Hawley D, Iversen SD. The selective CCK-B receptor antagonist L365,260 enhances morphine analgesia and prevents morphine tolerance in the rat, pp. 35-44, Copyright (1990), with permission from Elsevier.)

after surgery, treatment was commenced with saline, L365,260 or morphine alone or the combination of L365,260 and morphine. Behavioral testing was undertaken with vocalization threshold to paw pressure as the measure of antinociception. Acute doses of morphine were given. By day 16, baseline vocalization thresholds to paw pressure were the same in all four treatment groups, suggesting that pretreatment had no effect on the development of mechanical allodynia. Pretreatment with morphine alone twice daily for four days induced a complete tolerance to the antinociceptive effect of acute morphine. However, pretreatment with L365,260 and morphine completely prevented the development of tolerance to the antinociceptive effects of acute intravenous morphine. In this group, the effect of acute morphine was dose dependent, naloxone reversible, and similar to the effect of acute morphine seen in the saline-pretreated group.[6]

The majority of the work that examines the effect of CCK antagonists on antinociceptive tolerance utilizes morphine as the opioid. In clinical practice, morphine is only one of a number of strong opioids which are used. In intensive care practice, infusions of the short-acting, strong opioid alfentanil are frequently used while remifentanil infusions can be used as part of a total intravenous anesthetic technique. Use of such short-acting opioids, such as remifentanil in humans can be associated with tolerance.[7] Similarly, infusions of short-acting, strong opioids in animals are also associated with antinociceptive tolerance.[8] In the case of N-methyl-D-aspartate (NMDA) antagonists, their use is associated with a block on development of antinociceptive tolerance with morphine, but not with fentanyl or other selective mu- or delta-opioid agonists.[9] Therefore, even if evidence exists that CCK antagonists reduce the onset of antinociceptive tolerance with morphine, one cannot automatically extend this to other opioids. Kissin and colleagues (2000) affirm the concept that CCK antagonists may reduce antinociceptive tolerance when opioids are used and this does in fact extend to opioids other than morphine. They studied the effect of continuous infusion of the short-acting mu-opioid agonist alfentanil in rats. After four hours infusion of alfentanil, these rats were almost completely tolerant to the antinociceptive effects of alfentanil, as judged with a rat tail-pressure type test. They also assessed the effect of concomitant administration of the mixed CCK A and B antagonist proglumide, and the CCK B antagonists CI988 and L365,260. After four hours, all CCK antagonists had reduced the extent of antinociceptive tolerance with both proglumide and CI988 attenuating acute tolerance by around 50 percent while L365,260 attenuated the tolerance by about 25 percent (Figure 11.2).[10]

The finding that proglumide was as effective as CI988 and more effective than L365,260 in attenuating antinociceptive tolerance to alfentanil is interesting. Proglumide is known to have a low receptor affinity and one would have assumed that the more specific CCK B antagonists also studied would have had a more profound effect.

So far, the evidence points to CCK antagonists reducing tolerance to the effects of opioids. The question arises as to the effect of CCK agonists. One such mixed CCK A and B agonist with high affinity for both receptors is caerulein.[11,12] Zarrindast and colleagues (1997) studied the effects of CCK agonists and antagonists on morphine-antinociceptive tolerance. They found, as others have done, after four days of treatment with morphine that the study mice had be-

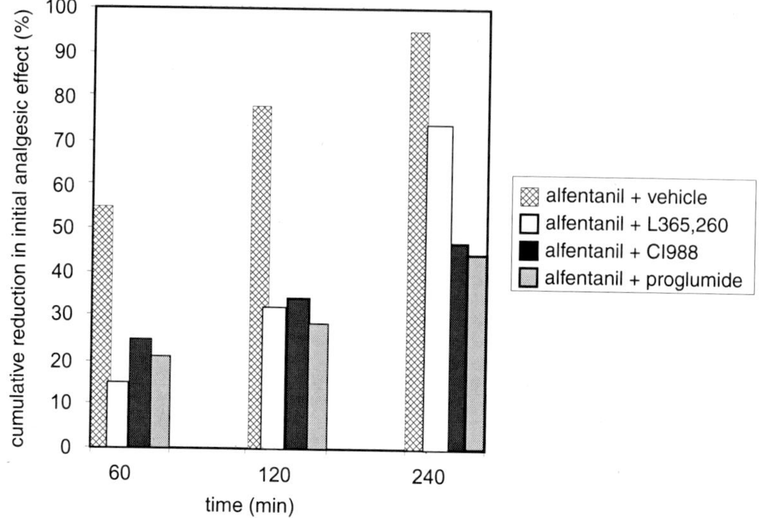

FIGURE 11.2. Comparison of the effects of CCK antagonists on acute tolerance to alfentanil-induced analgesia. Data presented as reduction in initial analgesic response. (*Source:* Kissin I, Bright CA, Bradley EL. Acute tolerance to continuously infused alfentanil: The role of cholecystokinin and N-methyl-D-aspartate-nitric oxide systems. *Anesth Analg* 2000; 91: 110-116. Reprinted with permission.)

come tolerant to its antinociceptive effects. If these animals were pretreated with caerulein prior to morphine administration for each of the four days, the antinociception produced by the morphine was potentiated. This potentiation produced by caerulein was reduced if the caerulein was administered with either MK329 or L365,260, both CCK antagonists. Furthermore, if either MK329 or L365,260 was given prior to morphine in the absence of caerulein, again antinociceptive tolerance was reduced.[13] They chose the hot-plate test as their nociceptive model. Others have shown that CCK-8 and caerulein cause antinociception when measured by the hot-plate test,[14,15] while the results when measured by the tail-flick test are less consistent.[16,17] In terms of the antinociceptive effect and the effect on antinociceptive tolerance produced by CCK agonists, among the variables that influence results are the species studied, antinociceptive test used, and the site of application of the agonist. In overall terms, the effects that CCK agonists have on antinociceptive tolerance give further weight to the argument that the CCK system is closely linked to the opioidergic system and that CCK has at least some influence on antinociceptive tolerance.

The same group went on to study whether the type of CCK agonist influenced the development of antinociceptive tolerance. As with other studies, tolerance to the effect of morphine quickly developed after daily morphine administration. Both caerulein and CCK-8 (which both have affinity for the CCK A and B receptors) decreased the development of antinociceptive tolerance to morphine. However, unsulphated CCK-8 (which has a low affinity for the CCK B receptor) had no such effect. As before, both the CCK A antagonist MK329 and the CCK B antagonist L365,260 also decreased the extent on antinociceptive tolerance to morphine. When CCK agonists and antagonists were coadministered, the effects on tolerance were dependent on the dose of antagonist used. Higher doses of MK329 caused a small decrease in attenuation of the morphine tolerance induced by CCK-8 and caerulein. Low doses of L365,260 diminished the effect of CCK-8 on morphine tolerance whereas high doses potentiated the response to caerulein. When animals were treated with MK329 or L365,260 before unsulphated CCK-8, reduction in tolerance to morphine was observed.[18]

The studies discussed so far consistently show that coadministration of a CCK antagonist with an opioid can reduce the extent or even prevent the onset of antinociceptive tolerance with repeated administration of that opioid. What if tolerance is already present? Hoffmann and Wiesenfeld-Hallin (1994) have shown that a CCK antagonist can indeed reverse established antinociceptive tolerance. They investigated the effect of the CCK B antagonist CI988 on tolerance to the antinociceptive effects of morphine in rats. After antinociceptive tolerance was induced by twice daily morphine administration for four days, the rats received either CI988 or saline, along with their usual morphine. In the saline group, tolerance was total. In those animals receiving CI988 with morphine, significant antinociceptive effect was observed.[19] This was not the first time that the ability to reverse established tolerance by the manipulation of the central CCK systems has been observed. When antiserum to CCK is administered intracerebroventricularly or intrathecally, established tolerance to morphine is reversed.[20] However, since antiserum does not cross the blood-brain barrier, this technique has little potential for human clinical use. We have seen already that proglumide also seems to reverse morphine tolerance.[1] However, whether this is actual reversal or is related to the delta-opioid-agonist properties of proglumide[21] and to the observation that chronic morphine administration causes an unregulation of delta-opioid-binding sites[22] is not firmly established. In contrast, CI988 has negligible affinity for mu-, delta-, or kappa-opioid receptors.[23] It could be argued that the apparent reversal of tolerance with CI988 could in fact be merely a potentiation of the morphine antinociception by the CI988. However, Hoffmann and Wiesenfeld-Hallin used a dose of CI988 that did not enhance the antinociceptive of morphine in morphine-naïve animals.

In an attempt to localize the area of the CNS in which CCK antagonists have their effect on antinociceptive tolerance, Tortorici and colleagues inserted catheters into the ventrolateral periaqueductal gray (PAG) of rats. They were able to induce antinociceptive tolerance to morphine within two days of repeated morphine administration into the PAG. However, if morphine administration was preceded by administration of proglumide applied to the same site, subsequent morphine always produced antinociception. When proglumide administration was stopped, tolerance soon developed. In morphine-tolerant rats, a single PAG injection of proglumide was enough to restore the antinociceptive effects of the morphine. If CCK was injected, a subsequent injection of morphine failed to elicit antinociception.[24] The findings in this study—that repeated microinjections of morphine into the PAG quickly results in tolerance is a consistent finding.[25,26] It may be that when morphine is systemically administered and subsequently reaches the PAG, it triggers local opioidergic circuits that trigger descending inhibition of nociception, and, on the other hand, induction of a local antiopioid action by CCK. This local induction of CCK would lead to tolerance.

In terms of the effect of morphine in the PAG, it has been suggested that it acts by inhibiting GABAergic neurones by reducing their release of synaptic GABA.[27] Such inhibition would eventually result in an enhanced activity of the output neurones of the PAG, which would then cause antinociception by directly or indirectly increasing the activity of the nociception-inhibiting "OFF" cells and decreasing the activity of the nociception-facilitating "ON" cells of the rostral ventromedial medulla.[26,28,29] "ON" and "OFF" cells project to the spinal dorsal horn[30] and are thought to mediate the PAG effect on nociception. CCK increases GABAergic activity,[31] which is the opposite of what opioids do in the PAG. Repeated administration of morphine may lead to induced hyperexcitability of PAG CCK-containing neurones and to increased drive of GABAergic neurones by CCK with consequent tolerance to further morphine administration.

The PAG is therefore important in the context of antinociceptive tolerance. Yet it is not the only site at which opioids have an effect and at which tolerance can be generated. In animals, repeated administration of an opioid in the presence of specific environmental cues induces tolerance specific to that setting. This is known as associative tolerance. Repeated administration of an opioid without consistent contextual pairing yields so-called nonassociative tolerance. Mitchell and colleagues (2000) produced associative tolerance in rats by administering morphine and saline in two distinct environments. After several administrations of morphine, further administration of morphine in the "morphine" environment failed to produce antinociception. However, if it was given to animals that had previously received morphine but the subsequent dose was given in the "saline" environment, full antinociception was apparent. The tolerance demonstrated is therefore "associative." Nonassociative tolerance was generated by implanting morphine pellets into the rats and administering saline in the environment used to condition the animals as in the associative-tolerance protocol. These animals rapidly became tolerant to morphine in all environments. They found that the CCK B antagonist L365,260, but not the CCK A antagonist MK329 blocked the expression of associative tolerance. Neither CCK antagonist affected the expression of nonassociative tolerance.

Mitchell and colleagues went on to determine the expression of Fos in associative- and nonassociative-tolerant animals. Animals who received morphine in the context of associative tolerance had significantly more Fos-positive cells in the lateral amygdala than those animals in the nonassociative tolerance groups. Increased expression of Fos was also observed in associatively tolerant animals in the basolateral amygdala and in area CA1 of the hippocampus. In contrast, no differences were found in other brain regions examined. When L365,260 was injected into the lateral or basolateral amygdala, associative tolerance was significantly attenuated. When injected into other areas, no such diminution is observed.[32] This suggests that CCK in the lateral and basolateral amygdala is required for the expression of associative tolerance to morphine and that the effect of CCK antagonists may be mediated by their action in these areas.

When taken in conjunction with the knowledge that CCK mRNA expression increases in the amygdala after repeated morphine administration,[33] the importance of the amygdala in the mechanisms involved in antinociceptive tolerance is emphasized.

CONCLUSIONS

The broadest conclusion that could be gained from this evidence is that CCK has a role in the onset of antinociceptive tolerance found with repeated administration of opioids. More specifically, a strong body of evidence gained from animal experimentation points to the ability of CCK antagonists to minimize and even prevent entirely the onset on antinociceptive tolerance with repeated dosing of opioids. Furthermore, if tolerance is already present, this can be easily reversed by CCK antagonist administration. In terms of associative tolerance, this seems to be generated by activation of CCK B in the amygdala. In overall terms, the periaqueductal gray seems also to be of major importance with chronic opioid use being associated with activation of CCK systems which influence the activity of "OFF" and "ON" cells in the rostral ventromedial medulla with their subsequent effects on the antinociceptive effects of the opioid.

A consistent finding in all the studies is the rapid onset of antinociceptive tolerance that occurs even after a few days of treatment with morphine or a few hours of treatment with alfentanil. In many cases, this tolerance is complete. Although it is not suggested that analgesic tolerance occurs as rapidly, or as completely in human practice, it would also be a stretch of the imagination to suggest that it does not occur at all. Even if it were accepted that analgesic tolerance does occur to a certain extent in human practice, any intervention that may minimize its effects or slow down the rapidity of its onset would be of clinical value. Yet CCK antagonists have not been studied in this context in humans.

In summary, the animal literature suggests that CCK antagonists reduce or even prevent the onset of antinociceptive tolerance with repeated opioid administration. Furthermore, if such tolerance is already present, they have the ability to completely reverse it.

Chapter 12

Is the Combination of Opioids and CCK Antagonists Safe?

So far, the evidence presented has almost uniformly confirmed that CCK acts as an antiopioid peptide whose levels are increased after neural injury and with chronic opioid use. Furthermore, opioid-derived antinociception can be increased by concomitant administration of a CCK antagonist and by so administering a CCK antagonist, antinociceptive tolerance associated with sustained use of opioids can be reduced or even eliminated. This evidence, all derived from animal experimentation, would at least suggest that CCK antagonists would be worth considering for use in human clinical practice.

Among the many side effects associated with strong opioid use, perhaps the most feared and acute is respiratory depression. It would not be unreasonable, therefore, to be cautious about coprescribing an agent that enhances the analgesic effect of the opioid used. Fortunately, two major pieces of evidence, one from work in squirrel monkeys, the other in humans, suggests that opioid-related side effects are not increased by coadministration of CCK antagonists.

L364,718 AND SQUIRREL MONKEYS

Dourish and colleagues studied the effects of the CCK A antagonist L364,718 (devazepide) on morphine-derived antinociception in a primate (squirrel monkey) model. Antinociception was measured using tail-withdrawal latency measurements in which the tails were put in cold and then hot water. As expected, L364,718, when administered alone had no antinociceptive effect. In contrast, morphine alone did produce a definite antinociceptive effect. When L364,718 and a similar dose of morphine were given together, an enhanced antinociceptive effect was observed. When larger or smaller doses of L364,718 were used with morphine, less enhancement was apparent, suggesting a bell-shaped dose-response curve[1]. The dose range over which effect was apparent was of the order of thirtyfold.

In a separate group of monkeys they administered morphine and measured respiratory rate, oxygen and carbon dioxide tension. As would be expected, morphine produced a dose-dependent decrease in respiratory rate and oxygen tension as well as an increase in carbon dioxide tension. When L364,718 was administered along with the same dose of morphine and at a dose that would have been expected to enhance morphine-derived antinociception, the changes in respiratory rate, oxygen and carbon dioxide tension were no different than that produced by morphine alone. Again, as would be expected, naloxone reversed completely the respiratory depression caused by the morphine. L364,718 use did not in any way compromise this effect[1] (Figure 12.1).

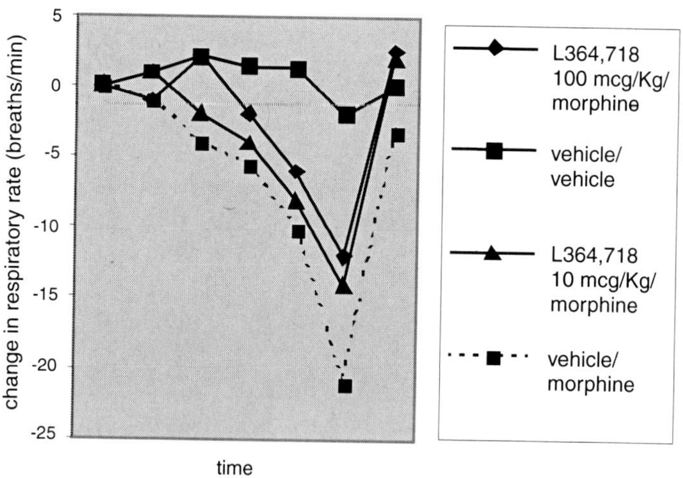

FIGURE 12.1. Effect of vehicle, morphine, L364,718 and L364,718 and morphine on respiratory rate in squirrel monkeys (naloxone given at last time interval). (*Source:* Reprinted with permission from Dourish CT, O'Neill MF, Schaffer LW, Siegl PK, Iversen SD. The cholecystokinin receptor antagonist devazepide enhances morphine-induced analgesia but not morphine-induced respiratory depression in the squirrel monkey. *J Pharmacol Exp Ther* 1990; 255: 1158-1165.)

This study suggests that the combination of a CCK antagonist and morphine produces no greater risk in terms of respiratory parameters than giving the morphine alone. It is also interesting from the perspective of the type of CCK antagonist studied. In the majority of animal studies CCK B antagonists seem to have the edge in terms of their ability to enhance morphine-derived antinociception. Most of these studies were performed in rodent or murine models. This is one of the few studies undertaken in a primate model showing that a CCK A antagonist very usefully enhanced morphine derived antinociception. This corresponds to the finding that CCK B receptors are the predominant type in rodents, while in the cynomolgus and squirrel monkeys the A type are more extensively represented.[2]

L365,260 AND HUMANS

Even with this reassuring evidence from a primate model, before CCK antagonist use could be contemplated in human practice, some assessment of its effect on opioid-related side effects in humans would be necessary. McCleane (2002) studied nine patients who were being treated with stable doses of sustained-release morphine for intractable neuropathic pain. Subjects were divided into three groups. Those in the first group were to receive two 10 mg doses of L365,260 with a four-hour gap between administrations. The second group received two 30 mg doses, while the last group received two 60 mg doses of L365,260. Serial measurements of electrocardiograms were made along with noninvasive blood pressure, heart rate, and respiratory rate. Subjects also recorded the occurrence and severity of side effects. Patients were studied for 24 hours in total. No significant alterations in any of the parameters measured, and in particular respiratory rate, were observed throughout the study period. A total of nine adverse effects were reported in five subjects. These were not serious and included dry mouth, bad taste, and headache.[3] As the study was an open-label study, it was hard to attribute these side effects to treatment rather than the study environment. The major focus of this small study was to address the more major safety concerns with the use of a combination of a CCK antagonist and strong opioid.

CONCLUSION

From the limited evidence available, there appears to be no acute enhancement of opioid side effects when a CCK antagonist is given along with that opioid. Indeed, if the CCK antagonist does enhance the opioid-derived analgesia, it may be possible to obtain the same level of pain relief with a smaller dose of opioid when a CCK antagonist is coadministered and expect a consequent reduction in the opioid-related side effects.

Chapter 13

Human Studies of the Combination of CCK Antagonists and Opioids

Although the many animal studies are of great interest and give an insight into the biological functions of CCK and help to understand the relationship between pain, and the opioidergic and CCK systems that influence pain, the real issue is whether the CCK antagonists have a role in human pain management. From the animal literature, one would expect that CCK antagonists would usefully enhance opioid-derived analgesia, reduce or prevent analgesic tolerance, and perhaps reverse established tolerance. Yet there are few human studies investigating this and no CCK antagonists currently licensed for use with opioids.

So, why are no CCK antagonists currently approved for use in human pain management? Does the evidence not support their use? Are there insufficient studies to define their effect? Or, could the lack of active patents put off investment in undertaking appropriate studies with a view to seeking approval? Many of the animal studies were carried out many years ago. Any patent protection has long since expired. The pharmaceutical industry is understandably reluctant to invest in appropriate studies needed to obtain approval. They would not be in possession of the intellectual property rights which would allow them to commercially exploit these agents, if found to be therapeutically active in this context.

In this chapter we will review the currently available human evidence on the effect of coadministration of CCK antagonists and opioids in a variety of experimental and clinical pain scenarios.

Cholecystokinin and Its Antagonists in Pain Management
© 2006 by The Haworth Press, Inc. All rights reserved.
doi:10.1300/5593_13

EXPERIMENTAL PAIN

One of the first human studies examining the effect of CCK antagonists on opioid analgesia was that of Price and colleagues (1985). They studied 80 volunteers who completed visual analogue scales to indicate their pain after a radiant heat was applied to the forearm. Temperatures of 45, 47, 49, and 51°C were delivered for a five-second interval to a 1cm^{2}area of skin. When 0.04 mg·kg^{-1} of morphine was given intravenously, no analgesic effect was apparent. When proglumide was given IV at a dose of 100 mcg alone or the combination of 0.04 mg·kg^{-1} morphine with 10 mcg proglumide, no analgesia was apparent. However, when 0.04 mg·kg^{-1} morphine was given with 100 mcg proglumide, a definite analgesic effect was apparent.[1] This combination of morphine and proglumide, (individually at a non-analgesic dose, but together with definite analgesic effect), produced analgesia that lasted for two hours, a time in excess of what would have been observed had morphine alone been used at a higher dose. The addition of 100 mcg proglumide to 0.04 mg·kg^{-1} produced analgesia the equivalent of approximately 0.08 mg·kg^{-1} morphine given alone, while the addition of 50 mcg proglumide to morphine 0.06 mg·kg^{-1} was equivalent to use of morphine 0.09 mg·kg^{-1}.[1] So, in this experimental situation, the addition of proglumide produced analgesia when morphine was used at a subanalgesic dose and this analgesia was of extended duration.

POSTSURGICAL PAIN

Dental Pain

Lavigne and colleagues (1989) used a third-molar-extraction dental-pain model to study the effect of proglumide on morphine-derived analgesia. They studied 60 patients who received intravenous morphine at a dose of 4 mg, 8 mg, and 4 mg with proglumide 0.05, 0.5, and 5 mg. Intravenous administration of 8 mg morphine alone was superior in terms of reduction in pain as measured on a visual analogue scale and duration of pain relief when compared to 4 mg alone. This 8 mg dose provided analgesia for 30 minutes. The 0.05 mg proglumide dose significantly enhanced the analgesic effect of morphine 4 mg and produced analgesia that was both more extensive and of significantly longer duration than that produced by morphine 8 mg alone (Figure 13.1). In contrast, the addition of proglumide 0.5 and 5 mg failed to enhance the effect of morphine.[2]

This enhancement of analgesia with proglumide was not accompanied by any observable increase in side effects beyond those seen when morphine was used alone. We have already seen that proglumide has a bell-shaped dose-response curve. In this study, it seemed that the lower dose of proglumide was most potent with the highest dose being superior to the intermediate dose. This biphasic response has also been observed in the rat tail-flick model.[3,4]

Abdominal and Gynacological Surgery

Lehmann and colleagues (1989) studied the effect of the mixed CCK A and B antagonist proglumide on the analgesic effect of morphine in patients who had undergone abdominal or major gynacological surgery. In the postoperative period, analgesia was provided

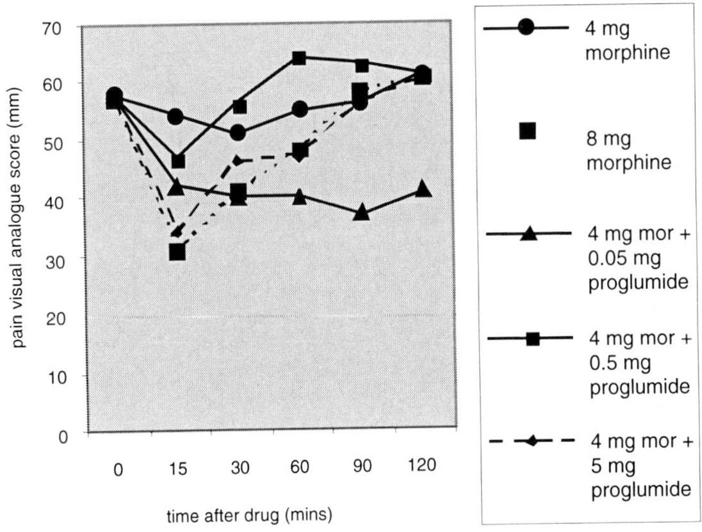

FIGURE 13.1. Effect of morphine alone and in combination with proglumide on dental pain. (*Source:* Reprinted from *Clin Pharmacol Ther,* 45, Lavigne GJ, Hargreaves KM, Schmidt EA, Dionne RA. Proglumide potentiates morphine analgesia for acute postsurgical pain, pp. 666-673, copyright 1989, with permission from American Society for Clinical Pharmacology and Therapeutics.)

with a patient-controlled analgesia system containing morphine. With this device, patients are required to press a button to receive a bolus dose of morphine, in this case 3 mg. A lockout period is programmed into the device so that after a successful administration of a bolus of morphine repeated depression of the button does not result in further morphine administration. In this study, the lockout period was two minutes. With these devices it is possible to establish not only the total morphine administration to a patient but also the hour-by-hour dose given. The 80 patients in this study were divided into four groups. The first received morphine only with all other groups receiving morphine and proglumide. Group two received 50 µg per 3 mg dose of morphine, group three 100 µg, and group four 50 mg proglumide. They also measured pain scores, and incidence of side effects. After 24 hours they found that there were no differences in the morphine consumption, pain scores, or incidence of side effects between the groups. The mean dose of morphine used by the patients was between 24 and 28 $\mu g \cdot kg^{-1}$ hr.[5]

The results of this study should be judged with some caution. The 80 patients studied were undergoing abdominal and major gynecological surgery. Those undergoing abdominal surgery were mostly cholecystectomies and gastric surgery whereas 19 out of the 21 patients having gynecological surgery had hysterectomies performed. Therefore, the range of surgery undertaken was wide. Even in those patients who had, for example, a cholecystectomy performed, we do not know if the operating surgeon was the same for all the cholecystectomies. Therefore, the nociceptive stimulus studied was potentially diverse ranging from a subcostal incision with the cholecystectomies to a suprapubic incision for the hysterectomies. A further concern is that the pain scores reported in this study were low from the start. At t = +1 hour, the average pain scores in all groups ranged from 1.0 to 1.6 on a 0 to 10 linear visual analogue scale. We do not know if the timing of measurement relates to the end of surgery, extubation, or the institution of the patient-controlled analgesia device. One wonders if local anesthetic was infiltrated in the wound or if a nonsteroidal anti-inflammatory accounts for the low pain scores, although neither intervention is mentioned in the study. The bolus dose of morphine used is also interesting. In this study, 3 mg was chosen. In clinical practice, it is more usual for this to be 0.5 to 2 mg. If a bigger bolus is used on a more infrequent basis, then the sensitivity of the results is diminished. Using a smaller bolus, which may, or may not result in the patient having to request an increase of morphine more frequently may have allowed a greater precision in the obtaining of results.

CANCER PAIN

To date, there is only one report of the use of a CCK antagonist and opioids in the field of cancer pain management. In this study, 60 patients with cancer pain who were being treated with opioids were enrolled. A crossover design was used. Forty-three patients completed both arms of the study protocol. A variety of opioids were being taken, including codeine, morphine, oxycodone, and buprenorphine. On study day one, patients were randomized to receive either their usual full dose of opioid alone with placebo or one-half of their usual dose along with proglumide 50 µg as their first analgesic dose of the day. The alternate dose was given at the midday dosing time (so those who received their full opioid along with placebo first thing now received half their normal opioid dose along with proglumide, and vice versa). On day two normal analgesia was given and on day three the order of treatment given on day one was reversed. Pain scores were recorded and side effects noted. No significant side effects were attributable to proglumide use. No changes in pain scores were recorded, suggesting that this small dose of proglumide was able to enhance the analgesic effect of the opioid to make up for half the dose being missed.[6] Clearly there is much difficulty in studying patients with cancer-related pain in view of the diversity of possible causes of pain and the ethics of withholding analgesia and hence the difficulty in carrying out placebo-controlled trials. One could conclude that this study gives a hint that proglumide was having some positive effect on opioid-derived analgesia, but there were only two single episodes in which proglumide was given and the duration of treatment was therefore much too short to allow definitive conclusions to be made. Interestingly, patients in this report were taking a wide variety of opioids and the effect with proglumide was not dependent on which opioid was being used. Two patients were taking buprenorphine whose principle effect is on the kappa receptor. For the results of this study to have meaning one would have to assume that halving a dose of an opioid for a single dose, set against a backdrop of regular opioid administration, and presumably the presence of steady-state levels of that opioid, would be manifest by an increase in pain. The lack of a third arm to this study in which half the normal dose of opioid would be given along with placebo, in place of proglumide, weakens the results somewhat, but then again the ethics of such a move in this patient group is questionable.

CHRONIC BENIGN PAIN

Evidence suggests that adding proglumide in a dose of 200 mg twice daily to extended-release morphine improves levels of pain relief without the imposition of extra side effects.[7]

McCleane (1998) studied 40 patients with intractable pain (neuropathic and nonneuropathic) who had been taking extended-release morphine at a stable dose. The average dose of morphine being taken was 50 mg per day with an average duration of use of around seven months. A crossover design was used with patients being treated with proglumide 200 mg twice daily for two weeks then placebo for two weeks or vice versa. At the end of the study period, median visual analogue scores had fallen in a nonstatistically significant fashion from 8 to 7 with placebo treatment, while with proglumide administration these scores had fallen in a statistically significant manner from 8 to 6. There were no significant differences in the incidence or severity of side effects between the placebo and proglumide treatment phases.[8]

The enhancement of analgesia with proglumide may also extend to other opioids. In a study of 30 adult patients with intractable pain who were treated with dihydrocodeine 60 mg twice daily, enhancement of analgesia was seen with proglumide administration. A crossover study design was used with subjects receiving proglumide 200 mg twice daily for two weeks followed by placebo twice daily for two weeks or vice versa. Pain was assessed by means of a 10 cm linear visual analogue scale. The mean pretreatment pain score was 8.12, with placebo treatment producing a mean pain score of 7.89. During the proglumide phase scores fell to 6.82. As before, side effects were not an issue with proglumide use.[9] Although the fall in pain scores was modest, they were achieved by coadministration of an agent that did not impose any extra side effects. Also, when proglumide was used in this and other studies, some subjects derived absolutely no extra relief while others had more marked, and even complete relief. The average pain scores with treatment fail to highlight the extent of relief gained by some.

NEUROPATHIC PAIN

A single case report suggests that proglumide can have an analgesic effect in patients with neuropathic pain when used alone.[10] In this case report, proglumide was used in a dose of 400 mg twice daily and the relief experienced by the cases in question was marked. No side effects were observed when proglumide treatment was initiated. The mechanism of this relief is not clear, but possibilities include the fact that proglumide exhibits delta-opioid-agonist activity[11] or that it was enhancing endogenous enkephalin-mediated analgesia, a phenomenon that has been demonstrated in animal models.[12-14]

To date, only one study has been reported investigating the effect of the more specific CCK A or B antagonists on opioid-derived analgesia in humans. McCleane (2003) studied the effect of the specific CCK B antagonist L365,260. Forty adult patients with chronic neuropathic pain unresponsive to currently available tricyclic antidepressants, antiepileptic drugs, nonsteroidal anti-inflammatories, and weak opioids were enrolled. All were taking stable doses of extended-release morphine, but deriving inadequate pain relief. Pain scores were recorded as a categorical pain rating (none, mild, moderate, severe) and utilizing a 10 cm linear visual analogue score. Measurements were taken for two weeks prior to study drug administration and for the remainder of the study period. All subjects received placebo, L365,260 30 mg, and L365,260 120 mg three times daily in divided doses in varying orders. Each treatment period was of two weeks, followed by a washout period of at least one week. Sleep and side effects were also assessed. At the end of the study period no differences were observed when baseline scores were compared to any of the active treatment phases. Nor was sleep altered, or serious adverse events recorded.[15]

The complete absence of any positive effect with L365,260 treatment has a number of possible explanations. First, the subjects enrolled were those who had failed to benefit from any previous therapeutic intervention and may have been too resistant to offer a fair test of the effect of L365,260. Second, as some of the subjects were able to observe benefit and correctly identify the active as opposed to placebo treatment phases, the pain-recording method may have lacked sensitivity. Third, L365,260 is a relatively weak inhibitor of spinal cord binding of CCK.[16] Fourth, as this is the first study in humans, incorrect doses may have been chosen. Fifth, the notion that CCK B antagonism may be more important in terms of opioid potentiation than CCK A may be incorrect. CCK A receptors are widely distributed in the cynomolgus monkey brain[16] in contrast to the more extensive representation of CCK B receptors in the rodents and mice[17,18] so perhaps a CCK A antagonist may have demonstrated some effect in contrast with the total lack of effect of this CCK B antagonist in this study. Although this study does suggest that L365,260 does not potentiate opioid analgesia in the patient group studied, the issue of analgesic tolerance and its ability to be influenced by CCK antagonists has not been addressed.

Unfortunately, to date, no published studies have investigated the effect of a CCK A antagonist on opioid analgesia in human subjects. Simpson and colleagues (2002) have presented an abstract of results from a study in patients with chronic neuropathic pain who were taking strong opioids in which the CCK A antagonist devazepide was investigated. In a double-blind, placebo-controlled crossover subjects were treated with placebo, devazepide 1.25 mg, and devazepide 5 mg given twice daily for two weeks each, separated by a washout period in varying orders. Simpson and colleagues reported, "devazepide significantly improved pain, activity and sleep scores compared to placebo" and "approximately 50 percent of patients reported pain relief with devazepide 5 mg."[19] Unfortunately, no further information in terms of pain scores, methodology, and outcome are given. Why this study has not yet been formally presented in the literature and exposed to peer review over four years after this abstract was published is a mystery.

ANALGESIC TOLERANCE

Despite the strong body of evidence in the animal literature suggesting that antinociceptive tolerance with opioids can be prevented or, if established, reversed by use of a CCK antagonist, the human literature is almost devoid of reports of investigation in this field.

Indeed, not all accept that analgesic tolerance is an issue with opioid use in humans and yet the animal studies show that antinociceptive tolerance occurs within hours if a short-acting, strong opioid is repeatedly administered, and within days if a longer-acting, strong opioid is used in a similar fashion.

McCleane (1998), in his crossover study of 40 patients taking extended-release morphine for chronic pain, reported that treatment with proglumide along with morphine provided better pain relief than when placebo was used with the same dose of morphine.[8] Of the 40 patients in this study, 13 elected, when blinding codes were broken, to remain on proglumide along with their usual dose of morphine. The baseline, pretreatment pain score in these 13 subjects was 8 and fell to 5.6 with proglumide treatment in that initial study. When followed up for one year, 10 of these 13 patients remained on the combination of morphine and proglumide. Their average pain scores, as measured by a 10 cm linear visual analogue scale were now 4.2.[20] Clearly, tolerance to the continued use of morphine had not occurred and indeed these subjects' pain levels had improved. This report gives a hint that analgesic tolerance with opioids can be minimized by use of proglumide, but of course the strength of evidence from this report is weak, given the small numbers and the lack of a placebo arm. This field merits further attention.

DIET AND ITS EFFECT ON ENDOGENOUS CCK LEVELS

CCK expression increases as a result of neural injury and chronic opioid administration. However, CCK is also released from the gastrointestinal tract on stimulation and has effects on the stomach, pancreas, and gallbladder. Although in many animal species the predominant alimentary form of CCK is the A variety with CCK being more important in terms of nociception, the picture may differ in primates and humans with CCK A having a greater central nervous system representation and importance in nociception.

Pahl and colleagues (2003) report their study on the effect of various liquid diets on pain perception and efficacy of opioids in a human model of acute pain and hyperalgesia. They found that a long-chain fatty-acid diet induced higher CCK release into the plasma than a diet containing medium-chain fatty acids. After diet administration, CCK levels rose after fifteen minutes and remained elevated for around fifteen minutes. When a long-chain fatty-acid diet was given during alfentanil infusion, the rise in plasma CCK levels was delayed, but were longer lasting. They assessed effects on pain perception and analgesia by using an electrical stimulation to a standardized area of the forearm and asking the subjects to rate their pain using an 11-point numerical rating scale. Hyperalgesia was measured using von Frey filaments and touch-evoked allodynia with a cotton-wool tip stroked against the skin. No effects from use of the liquid diets were observed in either the electrical stimulation pain test or on secondary hyperalgesia and the analgesic effects of alfentanil were unaltered by diet administration.[21] In this study, CCK-8 was measured and this has both CCK A and B activity. So despite an increase in plasma CCK levels, no effects were observed in terms of pain perception or response to an opioid analgesic. What is still not clear is the extent to which peripherally released CCK crosses the blood-brain barrier in humans. Zhu and colleagues (1986) have shown that in dogs CCK-33/39 and CCK-8 do not penetrate the blood-cerebrospinal fluid barrier in dogs,[22] but what effect a sustained increase in peripheral plasma CCK levels induced by a particular diet may have on the long-term penetration into the CSF is still not known.

This study does give some reassurance that for the population most likely to be using strong opioids, that is, those with a terminal disease who often have nutritional problems, alterations in diet probably do not influence their pain or response to opioids.

ISSUES WITH THE HUMAN LITERATURE

The following are some of the issues associated with the studies in the human literature.

- Low number of studies
- Whether CCK A or CCK B antagonist are most efficacious in humans
- Lack of studies investigating effect of CCK antagonists on analgesic tolerance
- Wide range of doses quoted for proglumide (Table 13.1)
- Lack of studies that investigate effect of CCK antagonists on opioids other than morphine and dihydrocodeine

TABLE 13.1. Doses of proglumide used with opioids in published human studies.

Type of pain	Opioid	Proglumide dose	Analgesia
Experimental	morphine	10 µg	no[a]
	morphine	100 µg	yes[a]
Dental pain	morphine	0.05 mg	yes[b]
	morphine	0.5 mg	no[b]
	morphine	5 mg	no[b]
Cancer pain	various	50 µg	yes[c]
Chronic pain	morphine	200 mg	yes[d]
Neuropathic pain	morphine	200 mg	yes[e]
Chronic pain	dihydrocodeine	400 mg	yes[f]

Sources: [a]Price DD, von der Gruen A, Miller J, Rafii A, Price C. Potentiation of systemic morphine analgesia in humans by proglumide, a cholecystokinin antagonist. *Anesth Analg* 1985; 64: 801-806; [b]Lavigne GJ, Hargreaves KM, Schmidt EA, Dionne RA. Proglumide potentiates morphine analgesia for acute postsurgical pain. *Clin Pharmacol Ther* 1989; 45: 666-673; [c]Bernsetein ZP, Yucht S, Battista E, Lema M, Spaulding MB. Proglumide as a morphine adjunct in cancer pain management. *J Pain Sympt Manage* 1998; 15: 314-320; [d]McCleane GJ. The cholecystokinin antagonist proglumide enhances the analgesic effect of morphine in chronic benign nociceptive and neuropathic pain. *Pain Clinic* 1998; 11: 103 0- 8; [e]McCleane GJ. The cholecystokinin antagonist proglumide enhances the analgesic efficacy of morphine in humans with chronic benign pain. *Anesth Analg* 1998; 87: 1117-1120; [f]McCleane GJ. The cholecystokinin antagonist proglumide enhances the analgesic effect of dihydrocodeine. *Clin J Pain* 2003; 19: 200-201.

The range of proglumide doses quoted in the literature is puzzling. Studies show a positive effect in terms of potentiation of morphine analgesia with doses ranging from 50 µg to 400 mg and yet other studies describe lack of potentiation with doses ranging from 10 µg to 5 mg. Definitive dose-finding studies are needed. They are probably as necessary with the other CCK antagonists as well. It is puzzling why an agent such as proglumide, which has low affinity for both CCK A and B receptors,[23] appears to fairly consistently be effective in potentiating morphine analgesia, and yet an agent with a significantly higher affinity for the CCK B receptor appears to be completely ineffective. An opportunity to compare the effect directly between proglumide and both a specific CCK A and a CCK B antagonist would help understanding considerably.

CONCLUSIONS

The available literature concerning the effect of CCK antagonists on opioid analgesia in humans is incomplete and confusing. The greatest body of evidence suggests that proglumide can be effective in enhancing morphine analgesia, but the dose at which it is most effective is far from clear. Despite what would be expected from the animal literature, the single published study of the effect of a specific CCK antagonist, in this case the B antagonist L365,260, fails to show any benefit in terms of enhanced pain relief with its use with morphine.

A large body of evidence from the animal literature suggests that CCK antagonists can enhance opioid-derived antinociception and reduce or prevent antinociceptive tolerance when they are used with opioids, yet the quality of the human evidence remains generally inadequate. If the suggestions from the animal literature are correct, the use of a CCK antagonist with an opioid, be it a weak or strong opioid, may become routine as it may enhance analgesia, reduce tolerance, and yet not impose a significant risk to increasing the side effects. This justifies significant further investigation in the human clinical situation.

Chapter 14

Other Potential Uses
of CCK Antagonists

Although the main focus of this book is on the relationship between CCK and opioid-derived analgesia, CCK antagonists have other potential clinical uses, some of which are pain related and worthy of mention.

BILIARY COLIC

The original description of CCK was in relationship to its effects on the gastrointestinal system and in particular the gallbladder, pancreas, and stomach. On ingestion of protein and fatty acids, CCK is released and promotes gallbladder contraction.[1] Conversely, administration of a CCK A antagonist will decrease gallbladder contraction.[2-4] Loxiglumide is one such potent and selective CCK A antagonist. Malesci and colleagues (2003) studied 14 patients with biliary colic (but no acute cholecystitis) and randomly assigned them to receive either loxiglumide intravenously or the conventional treatment of the anticholinergic hyoscine. Pain was assessed using a 100 mm visual analogue scale. If patients failed to get at least 80 percent relief within 30 minutes of the initial injection, the same compound was administered again. Pain relief was both faster and of greater proportions in the loxiglumide group with 88 percent of patients in the loxiglumide getting pain relief within 20 minutes as opposed to only 47 percent in the hyoscine group, while after 30 minutes these percentages rose to 92 and 49 percent, respectively. No adverse effects were observed after either treatment.[5] If this small study is an accurate reflection of the effects of this CCK A antagonist on biliary colic, then this treatment may be superior to conventional therapy.

PANCREATITIS

Pancreatitis is a condition characterized by recurrent abdominal pain, malabsorption, and diabetes mellitus. The pain caused by chronic pancreatitis is notoriously difficult to treat with strong opioids giving, at best, incomplete pain relief. Because some patients develop pancreatitis as a result of alcohol abuse, the prospect of using strong opioids in individuals with potentially addictive personalities is not attractive. Many patients with pancreatitis become well known to their medical practitioners because of their incessant requests for further strong opioid treatment. If one were to be cynical, one could think that these patients have become opiate addicts and demand further opioid administration to satisfy their craving. On the other hand, the pain produced by pancreatitis is severe and only partially responsive to even strong opioid treatment, so perhaps what these patients really crave is adequate pain relief rather than specifically further opioid use.

CCK has an antiopioid effect. Various studies have shown that in patients with pancreatitis, plasma CCK levels may be decreased,[6,7] normal,[8] or increased.[9-12] What is clearer is that plasma CCK tends to be increased by stimulation to a greater extent in patients with chronic pancreatitis who have significant pain.[13,14] McCleane (2000) reports a single patient with severe abdominal pain associated with chronic pancreatitis who derived only partial and short-lived pain relief from parenteral opioids. Intravenous administration of 1,400 mg proglumide over 24 hours produced pain relief that persisted for five weeks. Seven subsequent infusions of the same dose of proglumide produced pain relief that ranged from three to seven weeks. On no occasion were any side effects noted either during or immediately after infusion of proglumide.[15] CCK levels were not measured in this patient and so no firm conclusion can be reached regarding the mechanism of the apparent pain relief.

Administration of CCK or one of its analogues in large doses induces acute pancreatitis.[16,17] In addition, injection of CCK has been shown to worsen morbidity and mortality in experimental acute pancreatitis.[18-20] CCK antagonists have been shown to be effective in reducing the effects of acute pancreatitis following caerulein injection,[21,22] but not, it seems after the more severe taurocholate-induced[23] or bile-induced[24] pancreatitis. Satake and colleagues (1999) showed in an animal model of acute pancreatitis that the CCK A antagonist loxiglumide improves survival rates and minimizes pathological changes usually seen with induced pancreatitis and suggest that loxiglumide may have both therapeutic and possibly prophylactic effects on acute pancreatitis caused by various experimental interventions.[25]

ANXIOLYSIS

When CCK is injected into the periaqueductal gray in animals, an anxiogenic effect is observed. If the animals are pretreated with the CCK B antagonist PD135,158, but not the CCK A antagonist lorglumide, this anxiogenic effect observed normally after CCK icro-injection is blocked. When CCK-8 is injected alone into the periaqueductal gray, Fos-like immunoreactivity is increased in several brain areas related to defensive behavior, including the periaqueductal gray, median and dorsal raphe nuclei, superior colliculus, lateral nuclei, medial hypothalamus, and medial amygdala. This effect is again prevented by pretreatment with PD235,158.[26]

In humans, administration of CCK-4 induces panic attacks in volunteers,[27] while similar administration to patients with panic disorder reproduces their panic symptoms.[28,29] Hendrie and colleagues (1993) studied the effects of CCK A and B antagonists on anxiety in a mouse model. They utilized the black/white exploration model of anxiety and studied the CCK A antagonist L364,718, the less potent CCK A antagonist L365,031, and the CCK B antagonist L365,260. They found that L364,718 had a clear anxiolytic profile and had an inverted U-shaped dose-response curve. L365,031 also exhibited anxiolytic activity, but this was less marked than with L364,718. In contrast, the CCK B antagonist L365,260 had no discernable anxiolytic activity.[30]

An anxiolytic effect associated with CCK antagonist use is again highlighted by the report of Hughes and colleagues (1990). In the study by Hendrie and colleagues (1993), CCK A antagonists had definite anxiolytic effect while the B antagonist had none. The results presented by Hughes and colleagues (1990) are in marked contrast. They studied the CCK B antagonists PD134,308 and PD135,158 and used the mouse black/white test, as in the previous study. Both CCK B antagonists had marked anxiolytic effects and there was no evidence of the development of tolerance to their anxiolytic effects. Neither was there any sign of withdrawal anxiogenesis when use was discontinued after seven days. Both CCK antagonists were able to suppress the withdrawal anxiogenesis and produce an anxiolytic effect in mice previously tolerant to diazepam. Furthermore, both CCK B antagonists were able to produce significant anxiolytic effect in the rat elevated-plus maze test and the rat social-interaction test. These effects were comparable in magnitude to those seen with diazepam, but were produced without the sedation associated with diazepam use.[31]

The relevance of anxiety to the interaction of opioids and CCK is increased by the knowledge that systemic treatment with morphine at low doses induces an anxiolytic effect[32] and that the opioid antagonist naloxone potentiates the anxiogenic effect of CCK.[33] Koks and colleagues (1999) have shown that at low dose, morphine produces an anxiolytic effect and that this effect is blocked by coadministration of naloxone. A CCK B agonist, BOC-CCK-4, induced anxiety, while the CCK B antagonist L365,260 had an anxiolytic effect. The combination of L365,260 and a subeffective dose of morphine caused an anxiolytic effect not seen when either drug was administered alone at that dose.[34]

The serotinergic system may be involved in the anxiolytic effect of CCK antagonists. Bickerdike and colleagues (1994) studied anxiety in rats. Administration of the CCK A antagonist devazepide consistently produced anxiolysis, while the CCK B antagonist CI988 only produced anxiolysis on an inconsistent basis. The CCK B antagonist failed to have any anxiolytic effect. The anxiolytic effect of devazepide was attenuated by the 5-HT reuptake inhibitors zimelidine and Wy27587 at doses which, if given alone, had no anxiolytic effect.[35] Further evidence for an association between CCK-induced anxiety states and 5HT is given by the knowledge that 5HT can increase CCK release in the cortex via $5HT_3$ receptor activation,[36] and that conversely, CCK-4 can potentiate 5HT release in the guinea-pig frontal cortex induced by exposure to the elevated plus test.[37] Furthermore, the $5HT_3$ antagonist ondansetron can block anxiety induced by the CCK agonist caerulein.[38]

It seems, therefore, that CCK agonists induce anxiety while CCK antagonists have an anxiolytic effect. In some mouse experiments the A antagonists are more effective, while in others the B antagonists are superior. Which is most important in humans is yet to be defined. One wonders about the effect on anxiety of CCK elevations caused by neural injury and chronic opioid administration in human clinical practice.

DEPENDENCE
AND WITHDRAWAL REACTIONS

Opioids

Perhaps one of the greatest impediments to the more extensive use of strong opioids in clinical practice is the fear of opioid dependence and consequent withdrawal reactions on cessation of that treatment. In a rat model, Lu and colleagues (2000) found that administration of the CCK agonist caerulein increased the incidence of naloxone-induced withdrawal symptoms and delayed the extinction of morphine-conditioned place preference in morphine-dependent animals. These signs of morphine withdrawal and formation of morphine-conditioned place preference were suppressed by treatment with L365,260, but not by the CCK antagonist MK329.[39] Lu and colleagues (2001) confirm these results, again showing that pretreatment with L365,260 significantly attenuates the onset of conditioned place preference with repeated morphine use. After 28 days of the end of morphine use alone, conditioned place preference completely disappeared, but returned after a single morphine injection. Again, this reemergence of conditioned place preference with a single morphine injection is blocked by L365,260, but not by MK329.[40]

Valverde and Roques (1998) also studied the aversive component of acute morphine withdrawal precipitated by naloxone administration. They chronically treated the study rats with morphine alone and in combination with the CCK A antagonist devazepide, the CCK B antagonists L365,260 and PD134,308, and the CCK-B agonist BC264. On precipitated withdrawal, L365,260 partially decreased place aversion, PD134,308 completely blocked this aversion, while devazepide and BC264 had no effect.[41] It seems that CCK B and its antagonists, at least in a rat model, are of importance in precipitated withdrawal reaction. The implications for the management of human opioid dependence and withdrawal reactions are obvious.

Benzodiazepines

When rats are exposed to chronic administration of diazepam for 12 days and then treatment is terminated, a withdrawal reaction is precipitated. This withdrawal reaction can be measured using an auditory startle reflex. On diazepam withdrawal, acute pretreatment with diazepam or the CCK B antagonist LY288,513 dose-dependently block the withdrawal-induced increases in the auditory startle response.[42] When diazepam withdrawal occurs, the number of CCK receptors and CCK mRNA levels in the cortex and hippocampus increase.[43,44]

This effect is not restricted to rodents. Mice also develop withdrawal reactions after cessation of diazepam treatment. CI988, a selective CCK B antagonist, when administered alone, has anxiolytic properties[45,46] and its use is not complicated by withdrawal reactions when it is discontinued. CI988 dose-dependently antagonizes the anxiety reaction precipitated by diazepam withdrawal.[47]

It is possibly not only on the anxiolytic effect of benzodiazepines that CCK antagonists may have their effect. Panerai and colleagues (1987) have shown that the CCK antagonist CR1409 potentiated the anticonvulsant effect of diazepam as well as its effects on motor performance and spontaneous motor activity.[48]

Ethanol

Wilson and colleagues (1994) examined the effect of a CCK B antagonist, CAM1028 on the tolerance to chronic ethanol administration. When this CCK antagonist was coadministered with ethanol, at certain doses it was able to reduce the extent of tolerance development.[49]

In terms of withdrawal reactions, when the CCK A antagonist CAM1481 is administered after cessation of chronic ethanol administration in rats and mice, no changes in anxiety levels, as judged by the elevated maze-plus test, are observed. However, when the CCK B antagonists CAM1028 or CI988 are administered in a similar fashion, significant reductions in ethanol withdrawal anxiety are observed[50] suggesting that, at least in rodent and murine models, CCK B has a role in the genesis of this anxiety.

In addition to this effect in reducing ethanol-withdrawal-induced anxiety, the CCK B antagonists CAM1028 and CI988, when used at appropriate doses, can reduce ethanol-withdrawal-related seizure activity, an effect not seen with the CCK A antagonist CAM1481.[51]

CONCLUSIONS

Earlier chapters have highlighted the importance of CCK and opioid-derived antinociception and the potential role of CCK antagonists in maximizing opioid-derived pain relief. Some other potentially useful effects of CCK antagonists have been mentioned in this chapter. Perhaps the pain-relieving effect in biliary colic and pancreatitis is of little surprise given the strong association between CCK and this region of the gastrointestinal tract. Chronic administration of opioid drugs is not uncommon in patients with chronic pain conditions and the prospect of being able to reduce opioid-withdrawal reactions by use of a CCK antagonist during a period of opioid-dose reduction is interesting. Furthermore, that CCK antagonist could magnify the analgesia produced even by this reduced dose of opioid.

Another common feature of patients with chronic pain conditions is an apparent heightened level of anxiety which further complicates treatment. Again, the prospect of a CCK antagonist, primarily being used for its pain-relieving effect, also reducing anxiety, would be worthy of consideration.

As with the evidence surrounding the use of CCK antagonists in pain management, the human evidence regarding the use of this class of agent in anxiety, withdrawal, and dependency to opioids, benzodiazepines, and ethanol does not come anywhere near to that emanating from the animal literature.

Chapter 15

Conclusions

A mass of evidence confirms the important role that cholecystokinin plays in both the gastrointestinal tract and central nervous system. Also, cholecystokinin has an important influence on the action of opioids in the central nervous system. That is not to say that its importance is greater or of more importance than any other compound or neural regulatory system in the CNS, but rather that it is a potentially useful therapeutic target to improve the quality of pain relief for patients. Indeed, given the appealing concepts of a potential for enhancing opioid-derived analgesia while at the same time reducing the risk of analgesic tolerance occurring, it is surprising that more human clinical effort has not been put into substantiation of the claims made in the animal literature. The frustration of utilizing potent analgesics with well-defined and frequent side effects when the possibility exists for maximizing analgesia and minimizing side effects by coadministration of a compound with little risk of inducing side effects by itself will be obvious. The lack of commercial development of CCK antagonists is almost certainly not related to the lack of animal evidence that would bolster such development, nor to the lack of a perceived market for agents with the potential benefit of the CCK antagonists. More likely, it is based on purely commercial considerations relating to intellectual property rights and patent protection that would be needed in order to profit from development.

The action of CCK on stimulating gallbladder contraction and affecting gastric secretion has been highlighted. The evidence describing a reduction in biliary colic with the use of CCK antagonists is not surprising and the evidence that indicates a pancreato-protective effect is interesting. Acute pancreatitis is a potentially devastating illness and any intervention that could lessen pancreatic damage must have appeal.

Cholecystokinin and Its Antagonists in Pain Management
© 2006 by The Haworth Press, Inc. All rights reserved.
doi:10.1300/5593_15

Our major focus, however, has been on the interaction of CCK and opioids. The use of strong opioids in clinical practice is becoming more frequent. Yet it could be argued that they are not universally effective, not always the wisest choice of therapeutic agent, and perhaps not an option due to long-term effects. Again, anything that could maximize effect and minimize dose should have a place in clinical practice. There seems little doubt that CCK does interact with the opioidergic system in vivo and that CCK has an antiopioid effect. Strong evidence suggests that the expression of CCK and its receptors are influenced by a number of factors that include neural injury and chronic opioid administration. A clear deduction from this would be that neural injury or chronic opioid administration could be associated with a reduction of the analgesic effect of an opioid initially with a further reduction with the passage of time. This may precipitate an increase in opioid dose, which further compounds the problem. The literature concentrates on the effect of neural injury or chronic opioid administration on the expression of CCK and its receptors in the CNS. In practice, however, neural injury, which may produce neuropathic pain, is often now an indication for the use of strong opioids. What effect these combined factors have on the CNS expression of cholecystokinin is not known.

In relationship to analgesic tolerance, the ease with which antinociceptive tolerance can be produced in animals after only a few days of regular treatment with morphine is striking. That this tolerance is complete is even more remarkable. It is hard to imagine that sustained use of either weak or strong opioids in human clinical practice is not associated with at least partial analgesic tolerance, although some would say that tolerance to the effects of strong opioids is not a significant danger or clinical problem. Human studies are lacking of sufficient duration and design to give a definitive guide as to the occurrence and extent of tolerance in human practice. Even if we assume that tolerance occurs to some extent, even if it is partial, then any intervention that could delay its onset or minimize its extent would be of immense clinical benefit.

Outside the field of pain management, it is apparent that CCK has an effect on anxiety, dependency, and withdrawal reactions. In animal models, use of particular CCK antagonists can reduce anxiety, minimize dependency, and reduce the withdrawal reaction associated with, for example, precipitate withdrawal of opioids that have previously been chronically administered. Again, good applications of these concepts can be used in human practice, particularly in the field of pain management where many patients have an anxiety state by virtue of their condition, medication consumed, and possibly by their elevated CCK levels. If a CCK antagonist could reduce this anxiety, minimize dependency, and reduce the severity of withdrawal reactions, then that too would be useful.

Some significant dilemmas exist. We cannot assume that just because the majority of studies suggest that cholecystokinin B receptor antagonists have the greatest propensity for enhancing opioid-derived pain relief and minimizing tolerance that these animal studies are directly applicable to humans. The isolated primate studies suggest that cholecystokinin A receptor antagonists may in fact be more important in primates, and by implication humans. Therefore, the first dilemma is which type of cholecystokinin antagonist, be it A, B, or mixed, would have the most chance of being of value in humans. The second dilemma is the dose of cholecystokinin antagonist to investigate in humans. For example, the human proglumide evidence uses doses that range from 10 µg to 1,400 mg. One assumes that use of drugs such as proglumide can be more dose refined than this. The third issue is why such suggestive evidence from animal experimentation has not been more fully followed up in human studies. Certainly commercial considerations may have influenced this lack of human investigation, but this tardiness is a reflection of the enormous and valuable pursuit of knowledge currently taking place and, by comparison, the paucity of human clinical investigation.

In conclusion, a significant body of evidence from the animal literature suggests: the representation of cholecystokinin and its receptors is increased by neural injury and chronic opioid administration, cholecystokinin acts as an antiopioid peptide, cholecystokinin antagonists can enhance opioid-derived antinociception, prevent antinociceptive tolerance, and even reverse established antinociceptive tolerance (Figure 15.1).

A weak body of evidence exists in human literature suggesting that the mixed cholecystokinin A and B receptor antagonist proglumide can enhance opioid-derived analgesia; the optimal dose to achieve this effect is unknown. A single study suggests that the specific cholecystokinin B receptor antagonist L365,260 has no effect on opioid-derived pain relief, but no other published human studies yet

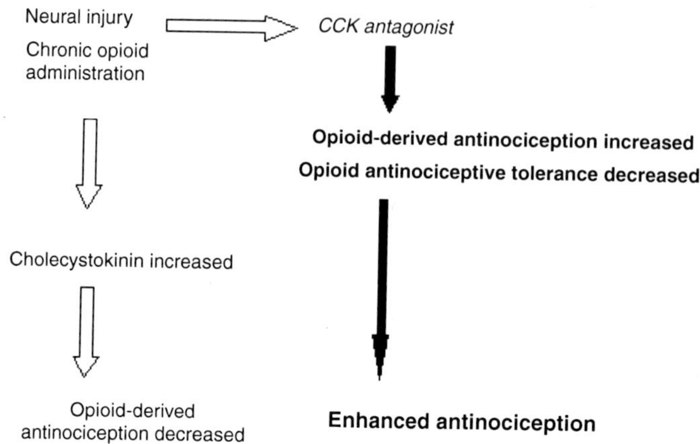

FIGURE 15.1. Proposed conclusions for effect of cholecystokinin and action of cholecystokinin antagonists in animal models.

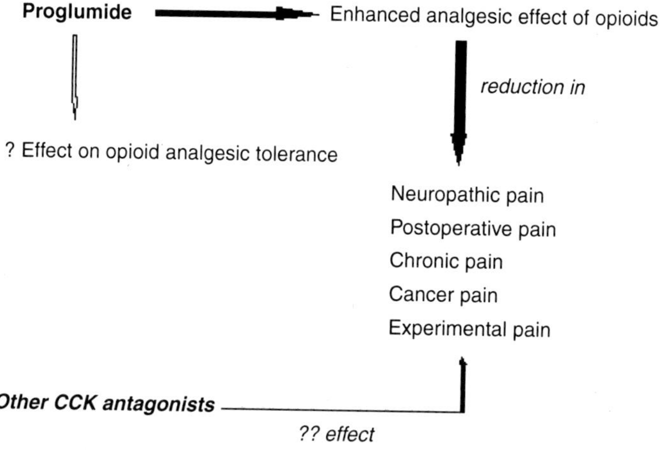

FIGURE 15.2. Summary of currently available information regarding the action of cholecystokinin receptor antagonists in human clinical practice.

exist that examine other cholecystokinin-receptor antagonists. Similarly, there are, as yet, no human studies that report the effect of any cholecystokinin receptor antagonists on opioid tolerance (Figure 15.2).

Notes

Chapter 2

1. Max MB, Byas-Smith MG, Gracely RH, Bennett GJ. Intravenous infusion of the NMDA antagonist, ketamine, in chronic posttraumatic pain with allodynia: A double-blind comparison to alfentanil and placebo. *Clin Neuropharmacol* 1995; 18: 360-368.

2. Rowbotham MC, Twilling L, Davies PS, Reisner L, Taylor K, Mohr D. Oral opioid therapy for chronic peripheral and central neuropathic pain. *N Eng J Med* 2003; 348: 1223-1232.

3. Inturrisi CE. Clinical pharmacology of opioids for pain. *Clin J Pain* 2002; 18: S3-13.

4. Gharagozlou P, Demirci H, Clarke JD, Lameh J. Activity of opioid ligands in cells expressing cloned mu opioid receptors. *BMC Pharmacology* 2003; 3: 1-8.

5. Narita M, Imai S, Itou Y, Yajima Y, Suzuki T. Possible involvement of mu1-opioid receptors in the fentanyl morphine-induced antinociception at supraspinal and spinal sites. *Life Sci* 2002; 70: 2341-2354.

6. Yamakura T, Sakimura K, Shimoji K. Direct inhibition of the N-methy-D-aspartate receptor channel by high concentrations of opioids. *Anesthesiology* 1999; 91: 1053-1063.

7. McDowell TS. Fentanyl decreases Ca^{2+} currents in a population of capsaicin responsive sensory neurons. *Anesthesiology* 2003; 98: 223-231.

8. Peloso PM, Bellamy N, Bensen W et al. Double blind randomized placebo control trial of controlled release codeine in the treatment of osteoarthritis of the hip or knee. *J Rheumatol* 2000; 27: 764-771.

9. Enggaard TP, Poulsen L, Arendt-Nielsen L et al. The analgesic effect of codeine as compared to imipramine in different human experimental pain models. *Pain* 2001; 92: 277-282.

10. Moore A, Collins S, Carroll D, McQuay H. Paracetamol with and without codeine in acute pain: A quantitative systematic review. *Pain* 1997; 70: 193-201.

11. Sindrup SH, Brosen K. The Pharmacogenetics of codeine Hypoalgesia. *Pharmacogenetics* 1995; 5: 335-346.

12. Williams DG, Patel A, Howard RF. Pharmacogenetics of codeine metabolism in an urban population of children and its implications for analgesic reliability. *Br J Anaesth* 2002; 89: 839-845.

13. Chew M, White JM, Somogyi AA, Bochner F, Irvine RJ. Precipitated withdrawal following codeine administration is dependent on CYP genotype. *Eur J Pharmacol* 2001; 425: 159-164.

14. Schmidt H, Vormfelde SV, Walchner-Bonjean M et al. The role of active metabolites in dihydrocodeine effects. *Int J Clin Pharmacol Ther* 2003; 41: 95-106.

15. Webb JA, Rostami-Hodjegan A, Abdul-Manap R et al. Contribution of dihydrocodeine and dihydromorphine to analgesia following dihydrocodeine administration in man: A PK-PD modelling analysis. *Br J Clin Pharmacol* 2001; 52: 35-43.

16. Schmidt H, Vormfelde S, Klinder K et al. Affinities of dihydrocodeine and its metabolites to opioid receptors. *Pharmacol Toxicol* 2002; 91: 57-63.

17. Raffa RB, Friderichs E. The basic science aspect of tramadol hydrochloride. *Pain Rev* 1996; 3: 249-271.

18. Wilder-Smith CH, Hill L, Spargo K, Kalla A. Treatment of severe pain from osteoarthritis with slow-release tramadol or dihydrocodeine in combination with NSAIDs: A randomised study comparing analgesia, antinociception and gastrointestinal effects. *Pain* 2001; 91: 23-31.

19. Silverfield JC, Kamin M, Wu SC, Rosenthal M. Tramadol/acetaminophen combination tablets for the treatment of osteoarthritis flare pain: A multicenter, outpatient, randomized, double-blind, placebo-controlled, parallel-group, add-on study. *Clin Ther* 2002; 24: 282-297.

20. Harati Y, Gooch C, Swenson M et al. Double-blind randomized trial of tramadol for the treatment of pain of diabetic neuropathy. *Neurology* 1998; 50: 1842-1846.

21. Boureau F, Legallicier P, Kabir-Ahmadi M. Tramadol in post-herpetic neuralgia: A randomized, double-blind, placebo-controlled trial. *Pain* 2003; 104: 323-331.

22. Sindrup SH, Andersen G, Madsen C, Smith T, Brosen K, Jensen TS. Tramadol relieves pain and allodynia in polyneuropathy: A randomised, double-blind, controlled trial. *Pain* 1999; 83: 85-90.

23. Sindrup SH, Madsen C, Brosen K, Jensen TS. The effect of tramadol in painful polyneuropathy in relation to serum drug and metabolite levels. *Clin Pharmacol Ther* 1999; 66: 636-641.

24. Adler L, McDonald C, O'Brien C, Wilson M. A comparison of once-daily tramadol with normal release tramadol in treatment of pain in osteoarthritis. *J Rheumatol* 2002; 29: 2196-2199.

25. Rowbotham MC, Reisner-Keller LA, Fields HL. Both intravenous lidocaine and morphine reduce the pain of postherpetic neuralgia. *Neurology* 1991; 41: 1024-1028.

26. Kalman S, Osterberg A, Sorensen J, Boivie J, Bertler A. Morphine responsiveness in a group of well-defined multiple sclerosis patients: A study with i.v. morphine. *Eur J Pain* 2002; 6: 69-80.

27. Attal N, Guirimand F, Brasseur L, Gaude V, Chauvin M, Bouhassira S. Effects of IV morphine in central pain: A randomized placebo-controlled study. *Neurology* 2002; 58: 554-563.

28. Caldwell JR, Rapoport RJ, Davis JC et al. Efficacy and safety of a once-daily morphine formulation in chronic, moderate-to-severe- osteoarthritis pain: Results from a randomized, placebo-controlled, double-blind trial and an open-label extension trial. *J Pain Symp Manage* 2002; 23: 278-291.

29. Maier C, Hildebrandt J, Klinger R et al. Morphine responsiveness, efficacy and tolerability in patients with chronic non-tumor pain—Results of a double-blind placebo-controlled trial (MONTAS). *Pain* 2002; 97: 223-233.

30. Hanks GW, Hanna M, Finlay I, Radstone J, Keeble T. Efficacy and pharmacokinetics of a new controlled-release morphine sulphate 200-mg tablet. *J Pain Symp Manage* 1995; 10: 6-12.

31. Walsh D, Tropiano PS. Long-term rectal administration of a high-dose sustained-release morphine tablets. *Support Care Cancer* 2002; 10: 653-655.

32. Wilkinson TJ, Robinson BA, Begg EJ, Duffull SB, Ravenscroft PJ, Schneider JJ. Pharmacokinetics and efficacy of rectal versus oral sustained-release morphine in cancer patients. *Chemother Pharmacol* 1992; 31: 251-254.

33. Fitzgibbon D, Morgan D, Dockter D, Barry C, Kharasch ED. Initial pharmacokinetic, safety and efficacy evaluation of nasal morphine gluconate for breakthrough pain in cancer patients. *Pain* 2003; 106: 309-315.

34. Roth SH, Fleischmann RM, Burch FX et al. Around-the-clock, controlled-release oxycodone therapy for osteoarthritis-related pain: Placebo-controlled trial and long-term evaluation. *Arch Intern Med* 2000; 160: 853-860.

35. Watson CP, Moulin D, Watt-Watson J, Gordon A, Eisenhoffer J. Controlled-release oxycodone relieves neuropathic pain: A randomized controlled trial in painful diabetic neuropathy. *Pain* 2003; 105: 71-78.

36. Watson CP, Babul N. Efficacy of oxycodone in neuropathic pain: A randomized trial in postherpetic neuralgia. *Neurology* 1998; 50: 1837-1841.

37. Oral oxycodone: New preparation. No better than oral morphine. *Prescrire Int* 2003; 12: 83-84.

38. Dellemijn PL, Vanneste JA. Randomised double-blind active-placebo-controlled crossover trial of intravenous fentanyl in neuropathic pain. *Lancet* 1997; 349: 753-758.

39. Soares LG, Martins M, Uchoa R. Intravenous fentanyl for cancer pain: A "fast titration" protocol for the emergency room. *J Pain Symptom Manage* 2003; 26: 876-881.

40. Bredenberg S, Duberg M, Lennernas B et al. In vitro and in vivo evaluation of a new sublingual tablet system for rapid oromucosal absorption using fentanyl citrate as the active substance. *Eur J Pharm Sci* 2003; 20: 327-334.

41. Bartfield JM, Flint RD, McErleane M, Broderick J. Nebulized fentanyl for relief of abdominal pain. *Acad Emerg Med* 2003; 10: 215-218.

42. Mystakidou K, Tsilika E, Parpa E et al. Long-term cancer pain management in morphine pretreated and opioid naïve patients with transdermal fentanyl. *Int J Cancer* 2003; 107: 486-492.

43. Menten J, Desmedt M, Lossignol D, Mullie A. Longitudinal follow-up of TTS-fentanyl use in patients with cancer-related pain: Results of a compassionate-use study with special focus on elderly patients. *Curr Med Res* Opin 2002; 18: 488-498.

44. Mystakidou K, Parpa E, Tsilika E et al. Long-term management of noncancer pain with transdermal therapeutic system-fentanyl. *J Pain* 2003; 4: 298-306.

45. Milligan K, Lanteri-Minet M, Borchert K et al. Evaluation of long-term efficacy and safety of transdermal fentanyl in the treatment of chronic noncancer pain. *J Pain* 2001; 2: 197-204.

46. Caplan RA, Ready LB, Oden RV, Matsen FA, Nessly ML, Olsson GL. Transdermal fentanyl for postoperative pain management. A double-blind, placebo study. *JAMA* 1989; 261: 1036-1039.

47. Ringe JD, Faber H, Bock O et al. Transdermal fentanyl for the treatment of back pain caused by vertebral osteoporosis. *Rheumatol Int* 2002; 22: 199-203.

48. van Seventer R, Smit JM, Schipper RM, Wicks MA, Zuurmond WW. Comparison of TTS-fentanyl with sustained-release oral morphine in the treatment of patients not using opioids for mild-to-moderate pain. *Curr Med Res Opin* 2003; 19: 457-469.

49. Larsen RH, Nielsen F, Sorensen JA, Nielsen JB. Dermal penetration of fentanyl: Inter- and intraindividual variations. *Pharmacol Toxicol* 2003; 93: 244-248.

50. Quigley C. Hydromorphone for acute and chronic pain. *Cochrane Database Syst Rev* 2002; 1: CD003447.

51. Bohme K. Buprenorphine in a transdermal therapeutic system—A new option. *Clin Rheumatol* 2002; 21: S13-S16.

52. Evans HC, Easthope SE. Transdermal buprenorphine. *Drugs* 2003; 63: 1999-2010.

53. Sittl R, Griessinger N, Likar R. Analgesic efficacy and tolerability of transdermal buprenorphine in patients with inadequately controlled chronic pain related to cancer and other disorders: A multicenter, randomized, double-blind, placebo-controlled trial. *Clin Ther* 2003; 25: 150-168.

54. Grilo RM, Bertin P, Scotto di Fazano C et al. Opioid rotation in the treatment of joint pain. A review of 67 cases. *Joint Bone Spine* 2002; 69: 491-494.

55. Quigley C. Opioid switching to improve pain relief and drug tolerability. *Cochrane Database Syst Rev* 2004; 3: CD004847.

56. Staats PS, Markowitz J, Schein J. Incidence of constipation associated with long-acting opioid therapy: A comparative study. *South Med J* 2004; 97: 129-134.

57. Milligan K, Lanteri-Minet M, Borchert K et al. Evaluation of long-term efficacy and safety of transdermal fentanyl in the treatment of chronic noncancer pain. *J Pain* 2001; 2: 197-204.

58. Menten J, Desmedt M, Lossignol D, Mullie A. Longitudinal follow up of TTS-fentanyl use in patients with cancer-related pain: Results of a compassionate use study with special focus on elderly patients. *Curr Med Res Opin* 2002; 18: 488-498.

59. Van Seventer R, Smit JM, Schipper RM, Wicks MA, Zuurmond WW. Comparison of TTS-fentanyl with sustained-release oral morphine in the treatment of patients not using opioids for mild-to-moderate pain. *Curr Med Res Opin* 2003; 19: 457-469.

60. Rowbotham MC, Twilling L, Davies PS, Reisner L, Taylor K, Mohr D. Oral opioid therapy for chronic peripheral and central neuropathic pain. *N Engl J Med* 2003; 348: 1223-1232.

61. Mystakidou K, Parpa E, Tsilika E et al. Long-term management of noncancer pain with transdermal therapeutic system-fentanyl. *J Pain* 2003; 4: 298-306.

62. Watson CP, Moulin D, Watt-Watson J, Gordon A, Eisenhoffer J. Controlled-release oxycodone relieves neuropathic pain: A randomized controlled trial in painful diabetic neuropathy. *Pain* 2003; 105: 71-78.

63. Schindler SD, Ortner R, Peternell A, Eder H, Opgenoorth E, Fischer. Maintenance therapy with synthetic opioids and driving aptitude. *Eur Addict Res* 2004; 10: 80-87.

64. Jamison RN, Schein JR, Vallow S, Ascher S, Vorsanger GJ, Katz NP. Neuropsychological effects of long-term opioid use in chronic pain patients. *J Pain Symptom Manage* 2003; 26: 913-921.

65. Tassain V, Attal N, Fletcher D et al. Long term effects of oral sustained release morphine on neuropsychological performance in patients with chronic non-cancer pain. *Pain* 2003; 389-400.

66. Sabatowski R, Schwalen S, Rettig K, Herberg KW, Kasper SM, Radbruch L. Driving ability under long-term treatment with transdermal fentanyl. *J Pain Sympt Mange* 2003; 25: 38-47.

67. Zacny JP, Gutierrez S. Characterizing the subjective, psychomotor, and physiological effects of oral oxycodone in non-drug abusing volunteers. *Psychopharmacology* 2003; 170: 242-254.

68. Grossman A. Brain opiates and neuroendocrine function. *Clin Endocrinol Metab* 1983; 12: 725-746.

69. Su CF, Liu MY, Li MT. Intraventricular morphine produces pain relief, hypothermia, hyperglycaemia and increased prolactin and growth hormone levels in patients with cancer pain. *J Neurol* 1987; 235: 105-108.

70. Paice JA, Penn RD, Ryan WG. Altered sexual function and decreased testosterone in patients receiving intraspinal opioids. *J Pain Symptom Manage* 1994; 9: 126-131.

71. Abs R, Verhelst J, Maeyaert J, Van Buyten J-P, Opsomer F, Adriaensen H, Verlooy J, Van Havenbergh, Smet M, Van Acker K. Endocrine consequences of long term intrathecal administration of opioids. *J Clin Endocrinol Metab* 2000; 85: 2215-2222.

72. Kokko H, Hall PD, Afrin LB. Fentanyl associated syndrome of inappropriate antidiuretic hormone secretion. *Pharmacotherapy* 2002; 22: 1188-1192.

73. Compton P, Athanasos P, Elashoff D. Withdrawal hyperalgesia after acute opioid physical dependency in non addicted humans: A preliminary study. *J Pain* 2003; 4: 511-519.

74. De Conno F, Caraceni A, Martini C, Spoldi E, Salvetti M, Ventafridda V. Hyperalgesia and myoclonus with intrathecal infusion of high-dose morphine. *Pain* 1991; 47: 337-339.

75. Heger S, Maier C, Otter K, Helwig U, Suttorp M. Morphine induced allodynia in a child with brain tumour. *BMJ* 319: 627-629.

76. Hood DD, Curry R, Eisenach JC. Intravenous remifentanyl produces withdrawal hyperalgesia in volunteers with capsaicin-induced hyperalgesia. *Anesth Analg* 2003; 97: 810-815.

77. Ossipov MH, Lai J, Vanderah TW, Porreca F. Induction of pain facilitation by sustained opioid exposure: Relationship to opioid antinociceptive tolerance. *Life Sciences* 2003; 73: 783-800.

78. Parisod E, Siddall PJ, Viney M, McClelland JM, Cousins MJ. Allodynia after acute intrathecal morphine administration in a patient with neuropathic pain after spinal cord injury. *Anesth Analg* 2003; 97: 183-186.

79. Sjogren P, Jensen N-K, Jensen TS. Disappearance of morphine induced hyperalgesia after discontinuing or substituting morphine with other opioid analgesics. *Pain* 1994; 59: 313-316.

80. Sjogren P, Jonsson T, Jensen N-K, Drenck N-E, Jensen TS. Hyperalgesia and myoclonus in terminal cancer patients treated with continuous intravenous morphine. *Pain* 1993; 55: 93-97.

81. Wolf CJ. Intrathecal high dose morphine produces hyperalgesia in the rat. *Brain Res* 1981; 209: 491-495.

82. Yaksh TL, Harty GJ, Onofrio BM. High dose of spinal morphine produce a non-opiate receptor mediated hyperaesthesia: Clinical and theoretical implications. *Anesthesiology* 1986; 64: 590-597.

83. Guignard B, Bossard AE, Coste C et al. Acute opioid tolerance: Intraoperative remifentanil increases postoperative pain and morphine requirement. *Anesthesiology* 2000; 93: 409-417.

84. Hood DD, Curry R, Eisenach JC. Intravenous remifentanil produces withdrawal hyperalgesia in volunteers with capsaicin-induced hyperalgesia. *Anesth Analg* 2003; 97: 810-815.

85. Devulder J. Hyperalgesia induced by high-dose intrathecal sufentanil in neuropathic pain. *J Neurosurg Anesthesiol* 1997; 9: 146-148.

86. Wang Z, Gardell LR, Ossipov MH et al. Pronociceptive actions of dynorphin maintain chronic neuropathic pain. *J Neurosci* 2001; 21: 1779-1786.

87. Vanderah TW, Gardell LR, Burgess SE, Ibrahim M, Dogrul A, Zhong C-M, Zhang E-T, Malan TP, Ossipov MH, Lai J, Porreca F. Dynorphin promotes abnormal pain and spinal opioid antinociceptive tolerance. *J Neurosci* 2000; 20: 7074-7079.

88. Vanderah TW, Ossipov MH, Lai J, Malan TP, Porreca F. Mechanisms of opioid induced pain and antinociceptive tolerance: Descending facilitation and spinal dynorphin. *Pain* 2001; 92: 5-9.

89. Vanderah TW, Suenaga NM, Ossipov MH, Malan TP, Lai J, Porreca F. Tonic descending facilitation from the rostral ventromedial medulla mediates opioid induced abnormal pain and antinociceptive tolerance. *J Neurosci* 2001; 21: 279-286.

90. Yaksh TL, Harty GJ. Pharmacology of the allodynia in rats evoked by high dose intrathecal morphine. *J Pharmacol Exp Ther* 1988; 244: 501-507.

Chapter 3

1. Ivy AC, Oldberg E. A hormone mechanism for gall-bladder contraction and evacuation. *Am J Physiol* 1928; 86: 599-613.

2. Boyden EH. Gall bladder contraction after blood transfusion. *Anat Rec* 1926; 33: 210.

3. Harper AA, Raper HS. Pancreozymin, a stimulant of the secretion of pancreatic enzymes in extracts of the small intestine. *J Physiol* 1943; 102: 115-125.

4. Mutt V, Jorpes JE. Structure of porcine cholecystokinin-pancreozymin. Cleavage with thrombin and with trypsin. *Eur J Biochem* 1968; 6: 156-162.

5. Jorpes E, Mutt VE. Cholecystokinin and pancreozymin: One single hormone? *Acta Physiol Scand* 1971; 66: 196-202.

6. Eysselein VE, Bottcher W, Kauffman GL, Walsh JH. Molecular heterogeneity of canine cholecystokinin in portal and peripheral plasma. *Regul Pept* 1984; 9: 173-185.

7. Fan ZW, Eng J, Miedel M, Hulmes JD, Pan YC, Yallow RS. Cholecystokinin octapeptides purified from chinchilla and chicken brains. *Brain Res Bull* 1987; 18: 757-760.

8. Maton PN, Selden AC, Chadwick VS. Large and small forms of cholecystokinin in human plasma: Measurement using high pressure liquid chromatography and radioimmunoassay. *Regul Pept* 1982; 4: 251-260.

9. Rehfield JF. Immunochemical studies on cholecystokinin. II. Distribution and molecular heterogeneity in the central nervous system and small intestine of man and hog. *J Biol Chem* 1978; 253: 4022-4030.

10. Mutt V. Cholecystokinin: Isolation, structure and function. In Glass GBJ (Ed.), *Gastrointestinal hormones*. New York: Raven Press 1989; 169-n203.

11. Dockray GJ, Vaillant C, Hutchinson JB. Immunochemical characterization of peptides in endocrine cells and nerves with particular reference to gastrin and cholecystokinin. In Grossman MI, Brazier MA, Lechago J (Eds.), *Cellular basis of chemical messengers in the digestive system.* New York: Academic Press 1981; 215-230.

12. Eberlein GA, Esselein VE, Goebell H. Cholecystokinin-58 is the major molecular form in man, dog and cat but not pig, beef and rat intestine. *Peptides* 1988; 9: 993-998.

13. Johnson AH, Rehfield JF. Identification of cholecystokinin / gastrin peptides in frog and turtle. *Eur J Biochem* 1992; 207: 419-428.

14. Frey P. Cholecystokinin octapeptide (CCK 26-33) nonsulfated octapeptide and tetrapeptide (CCK 30-33) in rat brain: Analysis of high pressure liquid chromatography (HPLC) and radioimmunoassay (RIA). *Neurochem Int* 1983; 5: 811-815.

15. Crawley JN, St-Pierre S, Gaudreau P. Analysis of the behavioural activity of C- and N- terminal fragments of cholecystokinin octapeptide. *J Pharmacol Exp Ther* 1986; 236: 320-330.

16. Innis RB, Synder SH. Cholecystokinin receptor binding in brain and pancreas: Regulation of pancreatic binding by cyclic and acyclic guanine nucleotides. *Eur J Pharmacol* 1980: 65: 123-124.

17. Sankaran H, Goldfine ID, Deveney CW, Wong KY, Williams JA. Binding of cholecystokinin to high affinity receptors on isolated rat pancreatic acini. *J Biol Chem* 1980; 255: 1849-1853.

18. Saito A, Goldfine ID, Williams JA. Characterization of receptors for cholecystokinin and related peptides in mouse cerebral cortex. *J Neurochem* 1981; 37: 483-490.

19. Jensen RT, Lemp GF, Gardiner JD. Interactions of COOH-terminal fragments of cholecystokinin with receptors on dispersed acini from guinea pig pancreas. *J Biol Chem* 1982; 257: 5554-5559.

20. Hays SE, Beinfeld MC, Jensen RT, Goodwin FK, Paul SM. Demonstration of a putative receptor site for cholecystokinin in rat brain. *Neuropeptides* 1980; 1: 53-62.

21. Praissman M, Martinez PA, Saladino CF, Berkowitz JW, Steggles AW, Finkelstein JA. Characterization of cholecystokinin binding sites in rat cerebral cortex using a ^{125}I-CCK-8 probe resistant to degradation. *J Neurochem* 1983; 1406-1413.

22. Dourish CT, Hill DR. Classification and function of CCK receptors. *Trends Pharmacol Sci* 1987; 8: 207-208.

23. Moran TH, Robinson P, Goldrich MS, McHugh PR. Two brain cholecystokinin receptors: Implications for behavioural actions. *Brain Res* 1986; 362: 175-179.

24. Mutt V. Further investigations of intestinal hormonal polypeptides. *Clin Endocr* 1976; 5: 175-183.

25. Deschenes RJ, Lorenz LJ, Haun RS, Roos BA, Collier KJ, Dixon JE. Cloning and sequence analysis of a cDNA encoding rat preprocholecystokinin. *Proc Natl Acad Sci USA* 1984; 81: 726-730.

26. Gubler U, Chau AO, Hoffman BJ, Collier KJ, Eng J. Cloned cDNA to cholecystokinin mRNA predicts an identical preprocholecystokinin in pig brain and gut. *Proc Natl Acad Sci USA* 1984; 81: 4307-4310.

27. Blanke SE, Johnsen AH, Rehfeld JF. N-terminal fragments of intestinal cholecystokinin—Evidence of release of CCK-8 by cleavage of the carboxyl side of arg (74) of proCCK. *Regul Pept* 1993; 46: 575-582.

28. Turkelson CM, Solomon TE, Hamilton J. A cholecystokinin metabolizing enzyme in rat intestine. *Peptides* 1990; 11: 213-219.

29. Deschodt-Lanckman M. Characterization of membrane-bound CCK-8 degrading enzymes from rat brain. *Arch Int Physiol Biochem* 1982; 90: 107-108.

30. Najdovski T, De Pont JJ, Tesser GI, Penke B, Martinez J, Deschodt-Lanckman M. Degradation of cholecystokinin octapeptide by the neutral endopeptidase EC 3.4.24.11 and design of proteolysis-resistant analogues of the peptide. *Neurochem Int* 1987; 10: 459-465.

31. Zuzel KA, Rose C, Schwartz JC. Assessment of the role of "enkephalinase" in cholecystokinin inactivation. *Neuroscience* 1985; 15: 149-158.

Chapter 4

1. Rehfeld JF. Immunochemical studies on cholecystokinin. II. Distribution and molecular heterogeneity in the central nervous system and small intestine of man and hog. *J Biol Chem* 1978; 253: 4022-4030.

2. Eng J, Shiina Y, Straus E et al. Post-translational processing of cholecystokinin in pig brain and gut. *Proc Natl Acad Sci USA* 1982; 79: 6060-6064.

3. Schultzberg M, Hokfelt T, Nilsson G et al. Distribution of peptide and catecholamine neurons in the gastrointestinal tract of the rat and guinea pig: Immunohistochemical studies using antisera to substance P, VIP, enkephalins, somatostatin, gastrin, Neurotensin and dopamine-B-hydroxylase. *Neuroscience* 1980; 5: 689-744.

4. Walsh JH, Lamers CB, Valenzuela JE. Cholecystokinin-octapeptide immunoreactivity in human plasma. *Gastroenterology* 1982; 82: 438-444.

5. Buffa R, Solcia E, Go VL. Immunohistochemical identification of the cholecystokinin cell in the intestinal mucosa. *Gastroenterology* 1976; 70: 528-532.

6. Buchan BM, Polak JM, Solcia E et al. Electron immunohistochemical evidence for the human intestinal I cells as source for CCK. *Gut* 1978; 19: 403-407.

7. Tsumuraya M, Nakajima T, Morinaga S et al. Morphological variation of immunoreactive cell positive to cholecystokinin-33 (10-20) and gastrin (1-15) in human duodenum. *Cell Tissue Res* 1986; 244: 519-525.

8. Hopman WP, Jansen JB, Lamers CB. Comparative study of the effects of fat, protein and starch on plasma cholecystokinin in man. *Scand J Gastroenterol* 1985; 20: 843-847.

9. McLaughlin J, Grazia-Luca M, Jones MN, D'Amato M, Dockray GJ, Thompson DG. Fatty acid chain length determines cholecystokinin secretion and effect on human gastric motility. *Gastroenterology* 1999; 116: 46-53.

10. Owyang C, Louie DS, Tatum D. Feedback regulation of pancreatic enzyme secretion: Suppression of cholecystokinin release by trypsin. *J Clin Invest* 1986; 77: 2042-2047.

11. Reimers J, Nauck M, Creutzfeldt W et al. Lack of insulinotropic effect of endogenous and exogenous cholecystokinin in man. *Diabetologia* 1988; 14: 271-280.

12. Go VL, Hoffman AF, Summerskill WH. Pancreozymin bioassay in man based on pancreatic enzyme secretion: Potency of specific amino acids and other digestive products. *J Clin Invest* 1970; 49: 1558-1564.

13. Liddle RA, Rushakoff RJ, Morita ET et al. Physiological role for cholecystokinin in reducing postprandial hyperglycaemia in humans. *J Clin Invest* 1988; 81: 1675-1681.

14. Becker HD, Werner M, Schafmayer A. Release of radioimmunologic cholecystokinin in human subjects. *Am J Surg* 1984; 147: 124-128.

15. Chen YF, Chey WY, Chang TM et al. Duodenal acidification releases cholecystokinin. *Am J Physiol* 1985; 249: 29-33.

16. Cantor P, Rehfeld JF. Cholecystokinin (CCK) in pig plasma: Release of components devoid of a bioactive COOH-terminus. *Am J Physiol* 1989; 256: 53-61.

17. Schaffalitzky de Muckadell OB, Olsen O, Cantor P et al. Concentrations of secretin and CCK in plasma and pancreatico-biliary secretion in response to intraduodenal acid and fat. *Pancreas* 1986; 1: 536-543.

18. Liddle RA, Goldfine ID, Rosen MS, Taplitz RA, Williams JA. Cholecystokinin bioactivity in human plasma: Molecular forms, responses to feeding, and relationship to gallbladder contractions. *J Clin Invest* 1985; 75: 1144-1152.

19. Konturek JW, Konturek SJ, Kurek A, Bogdal J, Olesky J, Rovati L. CCK receptor antagonism by loxiglumide and gallbladder contractions in response to cholecystokinin, sham feeding and ordinary feeding in man. *Gut* 1989; 30: 1136-1142.

20. Liddle RA, Gertz BJ, Kanayama S et al. Effects of a novel cholecystokinin (CCK) receptor antagonist, MK-329, on gallbladder contraction and gastric emptying in humans. *J Clin Invest* 1989; 84: 1220-1225.

21. Cantor P, Mortensen E, Myhre J et al. The effect of the cholecystokinin receptor antagonist MK-329 on meal-stimulated pancreaticobiliary output in humans. *Gastroenterology* 1992; 102: 1242-1251.

22. Gardner JD, Jensen RT. Secretagogue receptors on pancreatic acinar cells. In Johnson LR (Ed.), *Physiology of the gastrointestinal tract.* New York: Raven Press 1987; 2: 1109-1126.

23. Jensen RT, Lemp GF, Gardner JD. Interaction of cholecystokinin with specific membrane receptors on pancreatic acinar cells. *Proc Natl Acad Sci USA* 1980; 77: 2079-2083.

24. Jensen RT, Lemp GF, Gardner JD. Interactions of COOH-terminal fragments of cholecystokinin with receptors on dispersed acini from guinea pig pancreas. *J Biol Chem* 1982; 257: 5554-5559.

25. Sankaran H, Goldfine ID, Deveney CW, Wong KY, Williams JA. Binding of cholecystokinin to high affinity receptors on isolated rat pancreatic acini. *J Biol Chem* 1980; 255: 1849-1853.

26. Folsch UR, Cantor P, Wilms HM, Schafmayer A, Becker HD, Creutzfeldt W. Role of cholecystokinin in the negative feedback control of pancreatic enzyme secretion in conscious rats. *Gastroenterology* 1987; 92: 449-458.

27. Green GM, Lyman RL. Feedback regulation of pancreatic enzyme secretion as a mechanism for trypsin inhibitor-induced hypersecretion in rats. *Proc Soc Exp Biol Med* 1972; 140: 6-12.

28. Louie DS, May D, Miller P, Owyang C. Cholecystokinin mediates feedback regulation of pancreatic enzyme secretion in rats. *Am J Physiol* 1986; 250: G252-259.

29. Shiratori K, Shimuzi K, Watanabe S, Takeuchi T, Moriyoshi Y. Effect of CCK antagonists CR1409 and CR1505 on rat pancreatic exocrine secretion in vivo. *Pancreas* 1989; 6: 744-750.

30. Owyang C, Louie DS, Tatum D. Feedback regulation of pancreatic enzyme secretion-suppression of cholecystokinin release by trypsin. *J Clin Inv* 1986; 77: 2042-2047.

31. Hilderbrand P, Beglinger C, Gyr K et al. Effects of a cholecystokinin receptor antagonist on intestinal phase of pancreatic and biliary responses in man. *J Clin Inv* 1990; 85: 640-646.

32. Schmidt WE, Creutzfeld W, Schleser A et al. Role of CCK in regulation of pancreaticobiliary functions and GI motility in humans. Effects of loxiglumide. *Am J Physiol* 1991; 260: G197-206.

33. Adler G, Berlinger C, Braun U et al. Interaction of the cholinergic system and cholecystokinin in the regulation of endogenous and exogenous stimulation of pancreatic secretions in humans. *Gastroenterology* 1991; 100: 537-543.

34. Anika MS. Effects of cholecystokinin and caerulein on gastric emptying. *Eur J Pharmacol* 1982; 85: 195-199.

35. Chey WY, Hitanant S, Hendricks J, Lorber SH. Effect of secretin and cholecystokinin on gastric emptying and gastric secretion in man. *Gastroenterology* 1970; 58: 820-827.

36. Conover KL, Collins SM, Weingarten HP. A comparison of CCK-induced changes in gastric emptying and feeding in the rat. *Am J Physiol* 1988; 225: R21-26.

37. Debas HT, Farooq O, Grossman MI. Inhibition of gastric emptying as a physiological action of cholecystokinin. *Gastroenterology* 1975; 68: 1211-1217.

38. Dockray GJ. Mediation and modulation of gastric afferent function by regulatory peptides. In Tache Y, Wingate D (Eds.), *Brain gut interactions*. Boston: CRC 1991, 124-130.

39. Forster ER, Green T, Elliot M, Bremner A, Dockray GJ. Gastric emptying in rats. Role of afferent neurons and cholecystokinin. *Am J Physiol Gastrointest Liver Physiol* 1990; 258: G552-556.

40. Decktor DL, Pendelton RG, Elnitsky AT, Jenkins AM, McDowell AP. Effect of metoclopramide, bethanacol and the cholecystokinin receptor antagonist L-364,718 on gastric emptying in the rat. *Eur J Pharmacol* 1988; 147: 313-316.

41. Liddle RA, Gertz BJ, Kanayama S et al. Effects of a novel cholecystokinin (CCK) receptor antagonist, MK-329, on gallbladder contraction and gastric emptying in humans. *J Clin Invest* 1989; 84: 1220-1225.

42. Niederau C, Mecklenbeck W, Heindges T. Cholecystokinin does not delay gastric emptying of regular meals in healthy humans. *Hepatogastroenterology* 1993; 380-383.

43. Koop I, Dorn S, Koop H et al. Dissociation of cholecystokinin and pancreaticobiliary response to intraduodenal bile acids and cholestyramine in humans. *Dig Dis Sci* 1991; 36: 1625-1632.

44. Gomez G, Upp JR, Luis F et al. Regulation of the release of cholecystokinin by bile salts in dogs and humans. *Gastroenterology* 1988; 94: 1036-1046.

45. Koop I, Koop H, Gerhardt C, Schafmayer A, Arnold R. Do bile acids exert a negative feedback control on plasma CCK release? *Scand J Gastroenterol* 1989; 24: 315-320.

46. Schmidt WE, Creutzfeldt W, Hocker M et al. Cholecystokinin receptor antagonist loxiglumide modulates plasma level of gastro-entero-pancreatic hormones in man. *Eur J Clin Inves* 1991; 21: 501-511.

47. Koop I, Schindler M, Bosshammer A, Scheibner J, Stange E, Koop H. Physiological control of cholecystokinin release and enzyme secretion by intraduodenal bile acids. *Gut* 1996; 39: 661-667.

Chapter 5

1. Vanderhaegen JJ, Signeau JC, Gepts W. New peptide in vertebrate CNS reacting with antigastrin antibodies. *Nature* 1975; 257: 604-605.

2. Dockray GJ. Immunochemical evidence of cholecystokinin-like peptides in b rain. *Nature* 1976; 264: 568-570.

3. Innis RB, Snyder SH. Distinct cholecystokinin receptors in brain and pancreas. *Proc Natl Acad Sci USA* 1980; 77: 6917-6921.

4. Muller JE, Straus E, Yalow RS. Cholecystokinin and its COOH-terminal octapeptide in the pig brain. *Proc Natl Acad Sci USA* 1977; 74: 3035-3037.

5. Rehfeld JF. Immunochemical studies on cholecystokinin. II. Distribution and molecular heterogeneity in the central nervous system and small intestine of man and hog. *J Biol Chem* 1978; 253: 4022-4030.

6. Larsson LI, Rehfeld JF. Localization and molecular heterogeneity of cholecystokinin in the central and peripheral nervous system. *Brain Res* 1979; 165: 201-218.

7. Ju G, Melander T, Ceccatelli S, Hokfelt T, Frey P. Immunohistochemical evidence for a spinothalamic pathway co-containing cholecystokinin- and galanin-like immunoreactivities in the rat. *Neuroscience* 1987; 20: 439-456.

8. Hill DR, Woodruff GN. Differentiation of central cholecystokinin receptor binding sites using the non-peptide antagonists MK-329 and L365,260. *Brain Research* 1990; 526: 276-283.

9. Hill DR, Shaw TM, Graham W, Woodruff GN. Autoradiographical detection of cholecystokinin A receptors in primate brain using ^{125}I-Bolton Hunter CCK-8 and ^{3}H-MK-329. *J Neurosci* 1990; 10: 1070-1081.

10. Deschenes RJ, Lorenz LJ, Haun RS, Roos BA, Collier KJ, Dixon JE. Cloning and sequence analysis of a cDNA encoding rat preprocholecystokinin. *Proc Natl Acad Sci USA* 1984; 81: 726-730.

11. Savasta M, Palacios JM, Mengod G. Regional distribution of the messenger RNA coding for the neuropeptide cholecystokinin in the human brain examined by in situ hybridization. *Molec Brain Res* 1990; 7: 91-104.

12. Lindefors N, Linden A, Brene S, Sedvall G, Persson H. CCK peptides and mRNA in the human brain. *Progress Neurobiol* 1993; 40: 671-690.

13. Schiffmann SN, Vanderhaeghen JJ. Distribution of cells containing mRNA encoding cholecystokinin in the rat central nervous system. *J Comp Neurology* 1991; 304: 219-233.

Chapter 6

1. Wang X-J, Fan SG, Ren MF, Han S-J. Cholecystokinin octapeptide suppressed [³H]etorphine binding to rat brain opioid receptor. *Life Sci* 1989; 45: 117-123.

2. Wang X-J, Han J-S. Modification by cholecystokinin octapeptide of the binding of mu, delta and kappa opioid receptors. *J Neurochem* 1990; 55: 1379-1382.

3. Zhang X, Lucas GA, Elde R, Wiesenfeld-Hallin Z, Hokfelt T. Effect of morphine on cholecystokinin and mu opioid receptor like immunoreactivities in rat spinal dorsal horn neurons after axotomy and inflammation. *Neuroscience* 2000; 95: 197-207.

4. Wiesenfeld-Hallin Z, Xu X-J. Neuropeptides in neuropathic and inflammatory pain with special emphasis on cholecystokinin and galanin. *Eur J Phamacol* 2001; 429: 49-59.

5. Takashi M, Choitsu S, Munehiko N, Hogara N, Shigeaki B. G protein in stimulation of PI hydrolysis by CCK in isolated rat pancreatic acinar cells. *Am J Physiol* 1988; 255: 652-659.

6. Wang J, Ren M, Han J. Mobilization of calcium from intracellular stores as one the mechanisms underlying the antiopioid effect of cholecystokinin octapeptide. *Peptides* 1992; 13: 947-951.

7. Gustafsson H, Afrah A, Brodin E, Stillee C-O. Pharmacological characterization of morphine-induced in vivo release of cholecystokinin in rat dorsal horn: Effects of ion channel blockers. *J Neurochemistry* 1999; 73: 1145-1154.

8. Meunier JC, Mollereau C, Toll L et al. Isolation and structure of the endogenous agonist of opioid receptor-like ORL1 receptor. *Nature* 1995; 377: 532-535.

9. Reinschied RK, Nothacker HP, Bourson A et al. Orphanin FQ: A neuropeptide that activates an opioid like G protein-coupled receptor. *Science*1995; 270: 792-494.

10. Stanfa LC, Chapman V, Kerry N, Dickenson AH. Inhibitory action of nociceptin on spinal dorsal horn neurons of the rat. *Br J Pharmacol* 1996; 118: 1875-1877.

11. Candeletti S, Guerrini R, Calo G, Ferris S. Effect of the nociceptin receptor antagonist Phelps (CH2NH)-Gly2NC(1-13)NH2 on nociception in rats. 29th International Narcotic Research Conference. Garmisch-Partenkirchen, Germany, p. A170.

12. Carpenter KJ, Vithlani M, Dickenson AH. Unaltered peripheral excitatory action of nociceptin contrast with enhanced spinal inhibitory effects after carrageenan inflammation: An electrophysiological study in the rat. *Pain* 2000; 85: 433-441.

13. Maie IA, Dickenson AH. Cholecystokinin fails to block the spinal inhibitory effects of nociceptin in sham operated and neuropathic rats. *Eur J Pain* 2004; 484: 235-240.

14. Onaka T, Luckman SM, Guevara-Guzman R, Ueta Y, Kendrick K, Leng G. Presynaptic actions of morphine: Blockade of cholecystokinin-induced noradrenaline release in the rat supraoptic nucleus. *J Physiology* 1995; 482: 69-79.

15. Kendrick K, Leng G, Higuchi T. Noradrenaline, dopamine and serotonin release in the paraventricular and supraoptic nuclei of the rat in response to intravenous cholecystokinin injections. *J Neuroendocrinology* 1991; 3: 139-144.

16. Fujimoto JM, Schaus Arts K, Rady JJ, Tseng LF. Spinal dynorphin A (1-17): Possible mediator of antianalgesic action in mice. *Neuropharmacology* 1990; 29: 609-617.

17. Wang S, Rady JJ, Fujimoto JM. Elimination of the antianalgesic action of dynorphin A (1-17) by spinal transaction in barbital anesthetized mice. *J Pharmacol Exp Ther* 1994; 268: 873-880.

18. Rady JJ, Holmes BB, Fujimoto JM. Antianalgesic action of dynorphin A mediated by spinal cholecystokinin. *Proc Soc Exp Biol Med* 1999; 220: 178-183.

19. Vaught JL, Takemori AE. Differential effects of leucine and methionine enkephalin on morphine-induced analgesia, acute tolerance and dependence. *J Pharmacol Exp Ther* 1979; 208: 86-90.

20. Lee NM, Leybin L, Chang JK, Loh HH. Opiate and peptide interactions: Effect of enkephalins on morphine analgesia. *Eur J Pharmacol* 1980; 68: 181-185.

21. Barrett RW, Vaught JL. The effects of receptor selective opioid peptides on morphine-induced analgesia. *Eur J Pharmacol* 1982; 80: 427-430.

22. Vanderah TW, Lai J, Yamamura HI, Porreca F. Antisense oligodeoxynucleotide to the CCK B receptor produces naltrindole- and [Leu^5]enkephalin antiserum-sensitive enhancement of morphine antinociception. *NeuroReport* 1994; 5: 2601-2605.

23. Vanderah TW, Bernstein RN, Yamamura HI, Hruby VJ, Porreca F. Enhancement of morphine antinociception by a CCK B antagonist in mice is mediated via opioid delta receptors. *J Pharmacol Exp Ther* 1996;278: 212-219.

24. Fields HL, Vanegas H, Hentall ID, Zorman G. Evidence that disinhibition of brain stem neurones contributes to morphine analgesia. *Nature* 1983; 306: 684-686.

25. Heinricher MM, Morgan MM, Fields HL. Disinhibition of off-cells and antinociception produced by an opioid action within the rostral ventromedial medulla. *Neuroscience* 1994; 63: 279-288.

26. Benderson JB, Fileds HL, Barbaro NM. Hyperalgesia during naloxone-precipitated withdrawal from morphine is associated with increased on-cell activity in the rostral ventromedial medulla. *Somatosen Mot Res* 1990; 7: 185-203.

27. Pan Z, Hirakawa N, Fields HL. A cellular mechanism for the bidirectional pain-modulating actions of orphanin FQ/nociceptin. *Neuron* 2000; 26: 515-522.

28. Gao K, Chen DO, Genzen JR, Mason P. Activation of serotinergic neurons in the raphe magnus is not necessary for morphine analgesia. *J Neurosci* 1998; 18: 1860-1868.

29. Heinricher MM, McGaraughty S, Tortorici V. Circuitry underlying antiopioid actions of cholecystokinin within the rostral ventromedial medulla. *J Neurophysiol* 2001; 85: 280-286.

30. Hokfelt T, Rehfeld JF, Skirboll L, Ivemark B, Goldstein M, Markey K. Evidence for coexistence of dopamine and CCK in mesolimbic neurons. *Nature* 1980; 285: 474-478.

31. Hokfelt T, Skirboll L, Rehfeld JF, Goldstein M, Markey K, Dann O. A subpopulation of mesencephalic dopamine neurons projecting to limbic areas containing a cholecystokinin-like peptide: Evidence from immunocytochemistry combined with retrograde tracing. *Neurosci* 1980: 5: 2093-2124.

32. Gerhardt GA, Friedmann M, Brodie MS et al. The effects of cholecystokinin (CCK-8) on dopamine-containing nerve terminals in the caudate nucleus

accumbens of the anesthetized rat: an in vivo electrochemical study. *Brain Res* 1989; 499: 157-163.

33. Marshall FH, Barnes S, Hughes J, Woodruff GN, Hunter JC. Cholecystokinin modulates the release of dopamine from the anterior and posterior nucleus accumbens by two different mechanisms. *J Neurochem* 1991; 56: 917-922.

34. Ladurelle N, Keller G, Roques BP, Dauge V. Effects of CCK8 and of the CCK B selective agonist BC264 on extra cellular dopamine content in the anterior and posterior nucleus accumbens: A microdialysis study in freely moving rats. *Brain Res* 1993; 628: 254-262.

35. Hamilton ME, Freeman AS. Effects of administration of cholecystokinin into the VTA on DA overflow in nucleus accumbens and amygdala of freely moving rats. *Brain Res* 1995; 688: 134-142.

36. Beinfeld MC. What we know and what we need to know about the role of endogenous CCK in psychostimulant sensitization. *Life Sciences* 2003; 73: 643-654.

37. Fleetwood-Walker SM, Mitchell R, Hope PO, Maloney V, Iggo A. An alpha 2 receptor mediates the selective inhibition by noradrenaline of nociceptive responses of identical dorsal horn neurones. *Brain Res* 1985: 334: 243-249.

38. Sullivan AF, Dashwood MR, Dickenson AH. Alpha 2 adrenoreceptor modulation of nociception in rat spinal cord: Location, effects and interaction with morphine. *Eur J Pharmacol* 1987; 138: 169-177.

39. Sullivan AF, Kalso EA, McQuay HJ, Dickenson AH. The antinociceptive actions of dexmedetomidine on dorsal horn neuronal responses in the anaesthetized rat. *Eur J Pharmacol* 1992; 215: 127-133.

40. Sullivan AF, Hewett K, Dickenson AH. Differential modulation of alpha 2 adrenergic and opioid spinal antinociception by cholecystokinin and cholecystokinin antagonist in rat dorsal horn: An electrophysiological study. *Brain Res* 1994; 662: 141-147.

Chapter 7

1. De Mesquita MC, Beinfield MC, Crawley JN. Microdialysis as an approach to quantitate the release of neuropeptides. *Prog Neuropsychopharmacol Biol Psychiatry* 1991; 14: S5-15.

2. Wiesenfeld-Hallin Z, Lucas G de A, Alster P, Xu X-J, Hokfelt T. Cholecystokinin / opioid interactions. *Brain Res* 1999; 848: 78-89.

3. Xu X-J, Puke MJ, Verge VM, Wiesenfeld-Hallin Z, Hughes J, Hokfelt T. Upregulation of cholecystokinin in primary sensory neurons is associated with morphine insensitivity in experimental neuropathic pain in the rat. *Neurosci Lett* 1993; 152: 129-132.

4. Schiffman SN, Tengels E, Halleux P, Menu R, Vanderhaeghen JJ. Cholecystokinin mRNA detection in rat spinal cord motoneurons but not in dorsal root ganglia. *Neurosci Lett* 1991; 123: 123-126.

5. Schultzberg M, Dockray GJ, Williams RG. Capsaicin depletes CCK-like immunoreactivity detected by immunohistochemistry, but not that measured by radioimmunoassay in the rat dorsal root ganglia. *Brain Res* 1982; 235: 198-205.

6. Seroogy KB, Mohapatra NK, Lund PK, Rethelyi M, MacGehee DS, Perl ER. Species-specific expression of cholecystokinin messenger mRNA in rodent dorsal root ganglia. *Molec Brain Res* 1990; 7: 171-176.

7. Verge VM, Wiesenfeld-Hallin Z, Hokfelt T. Cholecystokinin in mammalian primary sensory neurons and spinal cord: In situ hybridization studies on rat and monkey spinal ganglia. *Eur J Neurosci* 1992; 5: 240-250.

8. Zhang X, Dagerland A, Elde RP et al. Marked increase in cholecystokinin B receptor messenger RNA levels in rat dorsal root ganglia after peripheral axotomy. *Neuroscience* 1993; 57: 227-233.

9. Ju G, Hokfelt T, Fischer JA, Frey P, Rehfeld JF, Dockray GJ. Does cholecystokinin-like immunoreactivity in rat primary sensory neurons represent calcitonin gene-related peptide? *Neurosci Lett* 1986; 68: 305-310.

10. Gustafsson H, Lucas G de A, Schott E et al. Peripheral axotomy influences the in vivo release of cholecystokinin in the spinal cord dorsal horn—Possible involvement of cholecystokinin B receptors. *Brain Res* 1998: 141-150.

11. Bras JM, Laporte A-M, Benoliel JJ et al. Effects of peripheral axotomy on cholecystokinin neurotransmission in the rat spinal cord. *J Neurochem* 1999; 72: 858-867.

12. Xu X-J, Alster P, Wu W-P, Hao J-X, Wiesenfeld-Hallin Z. Increased level of cholecystokinin in cerebrospinal fluid is associated with chronic pain-like behaviour in spinally injured rats. *Peptides* 2001; 22: 1305-1308.

13. Yaksh TL, Furui T, Kanawata IS, Go VL. Release of cholecystokinin from rat cerebral cortex in vivo: Role of GABA and glutamate receptor systems. *Brain Res* 1987; 406: 207-214.

14. Ravovska A. Cholecystokinin-GABA interactions in rat striatum. *Neuropeptides* 1995; 29: 257-262.

15. Bonoliel JJ, Bourgoin S, Mauborgne A et al. GABA, acting at both GABA-A and GABA-B receptors, inhibits release of cholecystokinin-like material from the rat spinal cord in vitro. *Brain Res* 1992; 590: 255-262.

16. Wilson PR, Yaksh TL. Baclofen is antinociceptive in the spinal intrathecal space of animals. *Eur J Pharmacol* 1978; 51: 323-330.

17. Allard LR, Beinfeld MC. Vasoactive intestinal polypeptide (VIP) inhibits potassium-induced release of cholecystokinin (CCK) from rat caudate-putamen but not from cerebral cortex. *Neuropeptides* 1986; 8: 287-293.

18. Brog JS, Beinfeld MC. Cholecystokinin release from the rat caudate-putamen, cortex and hippocampus is increased by activation of the D1 dopamine receptor. *J Pharmacol Exp Ther* 1992; 260: 343-348.

19. Yaksh TL, Abay EO, Go VL. Studies on the location and release of cholecystokinin and vasoactive intestinal peptide in rat and cat spinal cord. *Brain Res* 1982; 242: 279-290.

20. Nielsch U, Keen P. Reciprocal regulation of tachykinin- and vasoactive intestinal peptide-gene expression in rat sensory neurons following cut and crush injury. *Brain Res* 1989; 481; 25-230.

21. Shehab SA, Atkinson ME. Vasoactive intestinal polypeptide increases in areas of the dorsal horn of the spinal cord from which other neuropeptides are depleted following peripheral axotomy. *Exp Brain Res* 1986; 62: 422-430.

22. Zhou Y, Sun Y-H, Zhang Z-W, Han J-S. Increased release of immunoreactive cholecystokinin octapeptide by morphine and potentiation of mu-opioid analgesia

by CCK B receptor antagonist L-365,260 in rat spinal cord. *Eur J Pharmacol* 1993; 234: 147-154.

23. Ding XZ, Bayer BM. Increases of CCK mRNA and peptide in different brain areas following acute and chronic administration of morphine. *Brain Res* 1993; 625: 139-144.

24. Stanfa L, Dickenson AH. Cholecystokinin as a factor in the enhanced potency of spinal morphine following carrageenin inflammation. *Br J Pharmacol* 1993; 108: 967-973.

25. Zhang X, Lucas G de A, Elde R, Wiesenfeld-Hallin Z, Hokfelt T. Effect of morphine on cholecystokinin and mu-opioid receptor-like immunoreactivities in rat spinal dorsal horn neurons after peripheral axotomy and inflammation. *Neuroscience* 2000; 95: 197-207.

Chapter 8

1. Watkins LR, Cobelli DA, Faris P, Aceto MD, Mayer DJ. Opiate vs non-opiate footshock-induced analgesia (FSIA): The body region shocked is a critical factor. *Brain Res* 1982; 243: 119.

2. Faris PL, Komisaruk BR, Watkins LR, Mayer DJ. Evidence for the neuropeptide cholecystokinin as an antagonist of opiate analgesia. *Science* 1983; 219: 310-312.

3. Watkins LR, Cobelli DA, Mayer DJ. Opiate vs non-opiate footshock induced analgesia (FSIA): Descending and intraspinal components. *Brain Res* 1982; 242: 309.

4. Schafer M, Zhou L, Stein C. Cholecystokinin inhibits peripheral opioid analgesia in inflamed tissue. *Neuroscience* 1998; 82: 603-611.

5. Noble F, Smadja C, Roques BP. Role of endogenous cholecystokinin in the facilitation of mu-mediated antinociception by delta-opioid agonists. *J Pharmacol Exp Ther* 1994; 271: 1127-1134.

6. Noble F, Derrien M, Roques BP. Modulation of opioid antinociception by CCK at a supraspinal level: evidence of regulatory mechanisms between CCK and enkephalin systems in the control of pain. *Br J Pharmacol* 1993; 109: 1064-1070.

7. Friedrich AE, Gebhart GF. Modulation of visceral hyperalgesia by morphine and cholecystokinin from the rat rostroventral medial medulla. *Pain* 2003; 104: 93-101.

8. Kovelowski CJ, Ossipov MH, Sun H, Lai J, Mallan TP, Porreca F. Supraspinal cholecystokinin may drive tonic descending facilitation mechanisms to maintain neuropathic pain in the rat. *Pain* 2000; 265-273.

9. Petrovaara A, Wei H, Hamalainen MM. Lidocaine in the rostroventromedial medulla and the periaqueductal gray attenuates allodynia in neuropathic rats. *Neurosci Lett* 1996; 218: 127-130.

10. Heinricher MH, McGaraughty S. CCK modulates the antinociceptive actions of opioids by an action within the rostral ventromedial medulla: A combined electrophysiological and behavioural study. Abstract. 1996 International Association for the Study of Pain World Congress, August, Vancouver, Canada.

11. Fields HL, Heinricher MH. Anatomy and physiology of a nociceptive modulatory system. *Phil Trans Roy Soc Lond* 1985; 308: 361-374.

12. Fields HL, Bry J, Hentall I, Zorman G. The activity of neurons in the rostral medulla of the rat during withdrawal from noxious heat. *J Neurosci* 1983; 3: 2545-2552.

13. Fields HL, Heinricher MH, Mason P. Neurotransmitters in nociceptive modulatory circuits. *Annu Rev Neurosci* 1991; 14: 219-245.

14. Jurna I, Zetler G. Antinociceptive effect of centrally administered caerulein and cholecystokinin octapeptide (CCK-8). *Eur J Pharmacol* 1981; 73: 323-331.

Chapter 9

1. Galeone M, Moise G, Ferrante F, Cacioli D, Casula PL, Bignamini AA. Double-blind clinical comparison between a gastrin-receptor antagonist, proglumide, and a histamine H$_2$ blocker, cimetidine. *Curr Med Res Opin* 1978; 5: 376-382.

2. Miederer SE, Lindstaedt H, Kutz K, Mayershofer R. Efficient treatment of gastric ulcer with proglumide (Milid) in outpatients (double blind trial). *Acta Hepatogastroenterol (Stuttg)* 1979; 26: 314-318.

3. Hahne WF, Jensen RT, Lemp GF, Gardner JD. Proglumide and benzotript: Members of a different class of cholecystokinin receptor antagonists. *Proc Natl Acad Sci USA* 1981; 78: 6304-6308.

4. Bignamini AA, Casula PL, Rovati AL. Pharmacokinetic approach to proglumide long-term activity. *Arzneimittelforschung* 1979; 29: 639-642.

5. Rezvani A, Stokes KB, Rhoads DL, Way EL. Proglumide exhibits delta opioid agonist properties. *Alcohol Drug Res* 1987; 7: 135-146.

6. Chang RS, Lotti VJ, Monaghan RL et al. A potent nonpeptide cholecystokinin antagonist selective for peripheral tissues isolated from Aspergillus alliaceus. *Science* 1985; 230: 177-179.

7. Wisner JR, Renner IG. Asperlicin, a nonpeptidal cholecystokinin receptor antagonist, attenuates sodium taurocholate-induced acute pancreatitis in rats. *Pancreas* 1988; 3: 174-179.

8. Houch DR, Nodeyka J, Zink DL, Inamine E, Goetz MA, Hensens OD. On the biosynthesis of asperlicin and the directed biosynthesis of analogues of Aspergillus alliaceus. *J Antibiot (Tokyo)* 1988; 41: 882-891.

9. Bock MG, DiPardo RM, Rittle KE et al. Cholecystokinin antagonists. Synthesis of asperlicin analogues with improved potency and water solubility. *J Med Chem* 1986; 29: 1941-1945.

10. Goetz MA, Monaghan RL, Chang RS, Ondeyka J, Chen TB, Lotti VJ. Novel cholecystokinin antagonists from *Aspergillus alliaceus*. I. Fermentation, isolation and biological properties. *J Antibiot (Tokyo)* 1988; 41: 875-877.

11. Liesch JM, Hensens OD, Zink DL, Goetz MA. Novel cholecystokinin antagonists from *Aspergillus alliaceus*. II. Structure determination of asperlicins B, C, D, and E. *J Antibiot (Tokyo)* 1988;41: 878-881.

12. Lotti VJ, Pendleton RG, Gould RJ, Hanson HM, Chang RS, Clineschmidt BV. In vivo pharmacology of L364,718, a new potent nonpeptide peripheral cholecystokinin antagonist. *J Pharmacol Exp Ther* 1987; 241: 103-109.

13. Hill DR, Woodruff GN. Differentiation of central cholecystokinin receptor binding sites using the non-peptide antagonists MK329 and L365,260. *Brain Res* 1990; 526: 276-283.

14. Chang RS, Lotti VJ, Chen TB, Kunkel KA. Characterization of the binding of [3H]-(+/-)-L364,718: A new potent nonpeptide cholecystokinin antagonist radioligand selective for peripheral receptors. *Mol Pharmacol* 1986; 30: 212-217.

15. Taniguchi H, Yazaki N, Endo T, Nagasaki M. Pharmacological profile of T0632, a novel potent and selective CCK A receptor antagonist, in vitro. *Eur J Pharmacol* 1996; 304: 147-154.

16. Fukamizu Y, Nakajima T, Kimura K et al. Biochemical and pharmacological profiles of loxiglumide, a novel cholecystokinin A receptor antagonist. *Arzneimittelforschung* 1998; 48: 58-64.

17. Otsuki M, Fujii M, Nakamura T et al. Loxiglumide. A new proglumide analog with potent cholecystokinin antagonistic activity in the rat pancreas. *Dig Dis Sci* 1989; 34: 857-864.

18. Setnikar I, Chiste R, Giacovelli G, Rovati LC. Pharmacokinetics and tolerance of repeated oral doses of loxiglumide. *Arzneimittelforschung* 1989; 39: 1454-1459.

19. Setnikar I, Chiste R, Makovec F, Rovati LC, Warrington SJ. Pharmacokinetics of loxiglumide after single intravenous or oral doses in man. *Arzneimittelforschung* 1988; 38: 716-720.

20. Makovec F, Bani M, Cereda R et al. Pharmacological properties of lorglumide as a member of a novel class of cholecystokinin antagonists. *Arzneimittelforschung* 1987; 37: 1265-1268.

21. Makovec F, Bani M, Chiste R, Revel L, Rovati LC, Setnikar I. Different peripheral and central antagonistic activity of a new glutaramic acid derivatives on satiety induced by cholecystokinin in rats. *Regul Pept* 1986; 16: 281-290.

22. Chang RS, Chen TB, Bock MG et al. Characterization of the binding of [3H]L365,260: A new potent and selective brain cholecystokinin (CCK-B) and gastrin receptor radioligand. *Mol Pharmacol* 1989; 35: 803-808.

23. Lotti VJ, Chang RS. A new potent and selective non-peptide gastrin antagonist and brain cholecystokinin receptor (CCK-B) ligand: L365,260. *Eur J Pharmacol* 1989; 162: 273-280.

24. Dunlop J, Brammer N, Evans N, Ennis C. YM022 [R-1-[2,3-dihydro-1-(2'-methylphenacyl)-2-oxo-5-phenyl-1H-1,4-benzodiazepin-3-yl]-3-(3-methylphenyl)urea]: An irreversible cholecystokinin type-B receptor antagonist. *Biochem Pharmacol* 1997; 54: 81-85.

25. Dunlop J. CCK receptor antagonists. *Gen Pharmacol* 1998; 31: 519-524.

26. Attoub S, Moizo L, Laigneau JP, Alchepo B, Lewin MJ, Bado A. YM022, a highly potent and selective CCKB antagonist inhibiting gastric acid secretion in the rat, the cat and isolated rabbit glands. *Fundam Clin Pharmacol* 1998; 12: 256-262.

27. Saita Y, Yazawa H, Honma Y, Nishida A, Miyata K, Honda K. Characterization of YM022: Its CCKB / gastrin receptor binding profile and antagonism to CCK-8 induced Ca $^{2+}$ mobilization. *Eur J Pharmacol* 1994; 269: 249-254.

28. Dourish CT, O'Neill MF, Coughlan J, Kitchener SJ, Hawley D, Iversen SD. The selective CCK-B receptor antagonist L365,260 enhances morphine analgesia and prevents morphine tolerance in the rat. *Eur J Pharmacol* 1990; 176: 35-44.

29. Semple G, Ryder H, Rooker DP et al. (3R)-N-(1-(tert-butylcarbonylmethyl)-2,3-dihydro-2-oxo-5-(2-pyridyl-1,4-benzodiazepin-3-yl)-N'-(methylamino)phenyl)urea (YF476): A new and orally active gastrin / CCK-B antagonist. *J Med Chem* 1997; 40: 331-341.

30. Hruby VJ, Agnes RS, Davis P et al. Design of novel peptide ligands which have opioid agonist activity and CCK antagonistic activity for the treatment of pain. *Life Sciences* 2003; 73: 699-704.

Chapter 10

1. Watkins LR, Kinscheck IB, Mayer DJ. Potentiation of morphine analgesia by the cholecystokinin antagonist proglumide. *Brain Res* 1985; 327: 169-180.

2. Bodnar RJ, Paul D, Pasternak GW. Proglumide selectively potentiates supraspinal mu$_1$ opioid analgesia in mice. *Neuropharmacology* 1990; 29: 507-510.

3. Zarrindast M-R, Samiee F, Rezayat M. Antinociceptive effect of intracerebroventricular administration of cholecystokinin receptor agonist and antagonist in nerve-ligated mice. *Pharmacol Toxicol* 2000; 87: 169-173.

4. Wiesenfeld-Hallin Z, Xu X-J, Hughes J, Horwell DC, Hokfelt T. PD134,308, a selective antagonist of cholecystokinin type B receptor, enhances the analgesic effect of morphine and synergistically interacts with galanin to depress spinal nociceptive reflexes. *Proc Natl Acad Sci USA* 1990; 87: 7105-7109.

5. Coudore-Civiale M-A, Courteix C, Fialip J, Boucher M, Eschalier A. Spinal effect of the cholecystokinin-B receptor antagonist CI-988 on hyperalgesia, allodynia and morphine-induced analgesia in diabetic and mononeuropathic rats. *Pain* 2000; 88: 15-22.

6. Xu X-J, Seiger A, Hughes J, Hokfelt T, Wiesenfeld-Hallin Z. Chronic pain-related behaviours in spinally injured rats: Evidence for functional alterations of the endogenous cholecystokinin and opioid systems. *Pain* 1994; 56: 271-277.

7. O'Neill MF, Dourish CT, Tye SJ, Iversen SD. Blockade of CCK-B receptors by L365,260 induces analgesia in the squirrel monkey. *Brain Res* 1990; 534: 287-290.

8. Nichols ML, Bian D, Ossipov MH, Lai J, Porreca F. Regulation of morphine antiallodynia efficacy by cholecystokinin in a model of neuropathic pain in rats. *J Pharmacol Exp Ther* 1995; 275: 1339-1345.

9. Yamamoto T, Sakashita Y. Differential effects of intrathecally administered morphine and its interaction with cholecystokinin-B antagonist on thermal hyperalgesia following two models of experimental mononeuropathy in the rat. *Anesthesiology* 1999; 90: 1382-1391.

10. Friederich AE, Gebhart GF. Effects of spinal cholecystokinin receptor antagonists on morphine antinociception in a model of visceral pain in the rat. *J Pharmacol Exp Ther* 2000; 292: 538-544.

11. Lavigne GJ, Millington WR, Mueller GP. The CCK-A and CCK-B receptor antagonists, devazepide and L365,260, enhance morphine antinociception only in non-acclimated rats exposed to a novel environment. *Neuropeptides* 1992; 21: 119-129.

12. Dourish CT, Hawley D, Iversen SD. Enhancement of morphine analgesia and prevention of morphine tolerance in the rat by the cholecystokinin antagonist L364,718. *Eur J Pharmacol* 1988; 147: 469-472.

13. Dourish CT, O'Neill MF, Coughlan J, Kitchener SJ, Hawley D, Iversen SD. The selective CCK-B receptor antagonist L365,260 enhances morphine analgesia and prevents morphine tolerance in the rat. *Eur J Pharmacol* 1990; 176: 35-44.

14. Calcagnetti D-J, Holtzman SG. Factors affecting restraint stress-induced potentiation of morphine analgesia. *Brain Res* 1990; 537: 157-162.

15. Lichtman A, Fanselow MS. Cats produce analgesia in rats on the tail-flick test: Naltexone sensitivity is determined by the nociceptive test stimulus. *Brain Res* 1990; 533: 91-94.

16. Bushnell MC, Duncan GH, Dubner R, Jones RL, Maixner W. Attentional influences on noxious and innocuous cutaneous heat detection in humans and monkeys. *J Neurosci* 1985; 5: 1103-1110.

17. Suh HW, Kim Y-H, Choi YS, Song DK. Involvement of different subtypes of cholecystokinin receptors in opioid antinociception in the mouse. *Peptides* 1995; 16: 1229-1234.

18. Singh L, Oles RJ, Field MJ, Atwal P, Woodruff GN, Hunter JC. Effect of CCK receptor antagonists on the antinociceptive, reinforcing and gut motility properties of morphine. *Br J Pharmacol* 1996; 118: 1317-1325.

19. Yamamoto T, Nozaki-Taguchi N. The effects of intrathecally administered FK480, a cholecystokinin-A receptor antagonist, and YM022, a cholecystokinin-B receptor antagonist, on the formalin test in the rat. *Anesth Analg* 1996;83: 107-113.

20. Migaud M, Roques BP, Durieux C. Effects of cholecystokinin octapeptide and BC264, a potent and selective CCK-B agonist on aspartate and glutamate release from rat hippocampal slices. *Neuropharmacol* 1994; 33: 737-743.

21. Kellstein DE, Mayer DJ. Chronic administration of cholecystokinin antagonists reverses the enhancement of spinal morphine analgesia induced by acute pretreatment. *Brain Res* 1990; 516: 263-270.

22. Ruiz-Gayo M, Durieux C, Fournie-Zaluski MC, Roques BP. Stimulation of delta opioid receptors reduces the in vivo binding of the CCK-B selective agonist [^{3}H]pBC264: Evidence for a physiological regulation of CCKergic system by endogenous enkephalins. *J Neurochem* 1992; 59: 1805-1811.

23. Noble F, Soleilhac JM, Soroca-Lucas E, Turcaud S, Fournie-Zaluski MC, Roques BP. Inhibition of the enkephalin metabolizing enzymes by the first systemically active mixed inhibitor prodrug RB101 induces potent analgesic response in rats and mice. *J Pharmacol Exp Ther* 1992; 261: 181-190.

24. Valverde O, Maldonado R, Fournie-Zaluski MC, Roques BP. Cholecystokinin B antagonists strongly potentiate antinociception mediated by endogenous enkephalins. *J Pharmacol Exp Ther* 1994; 270: 77-88.

25. Coudore-Civiale MA, Meen M, Fournie-Zaluski MC, Boucher M, Roques BP, Eschalier A. Enhancement of the effects of a complete inhibitor of enkephalin-catabolizing enzymes, RB101, by a cholecystokinin B receptor antagonist in diabetic rats. *Br J Pharmacol* 2001; 133: 179-185.

26. Maldonado R, Valverde O, Ducos B, Blommaert AG, Fournie-Zaluski MC, Roques BP. Inhibition of morphine withdrawal by the association of RB101, an inhibitor of enkephalin catabolism, and the CCK B antagonist PD134,308. *Br J Pharmcol* 1995; 1031-1039.

27. Le Guen S, Nieto MM, Canestrelli C et al. Pain management by a new series of dual inhibitors of enkephalin degrading enzymes: Long lasting antinociceptive properties and potentiation by CCK$_2$ antagonist or methadone. *Pain* 2003; 104: 139-148.

28. Vanderah TW, Bernstein RN, Lai J, Porreca F. Production of naltrindole-sensitive antinociception by a cholecystokinin (CCK) antagonist and thiorphan: Evidence for tonic inhibition of enkephalin release by CCK. *Analgesia* 1995; 1: 813-816.

29. Coudore-Civiale MA, Courteix C, Boucher M et al. Potentiation of morphine and clomipramine analgesia by cholecystokinin-B antagonist CI988 in diabetic rats. *Neurosci Lett* 2000; 286: 37-40.

30. Van Megen HJ, Westenberg HG, den Boer JA, Slaap B, Scheepmakers A. Effect of the selective serotonin reuptake inhibitor fluvoxamine on CCK-4 induced panic attacks. *Psychopharmacology* 1997; 129: 357-364.

31. Biro E, Penke B, Telegdy G. Role of different neurotransmitter systems in the cholecystokinin octapeptide-induced anxiogenic response in rats. *Neuropeptides* 1997; 31: 281-285.

32. Ardid D, Guilbaud G. Antinociceptive effects of acute and "chronic" injections of tricyclic antidepressant drugs in a new model of neuropathy in rats. *Pain* 1992; 49: 279-287.

Chapter 11

1. Watkins LR, Kinscheck IB, Mayer DJ. Potentiation of opiate analgesia and apparent reversal of morphine tolerance by proglumide. *Science* 1984; 224; 395-396.

2. Tang J, Chou J, Iadarola M, Yang H-YT, Costa E. Proglumide prevents and curtails acute tolerance to morphine in rats. *Neuropharmacology* 1984; 23: 715-718.

3. Panerai AE, Rovati LC, Cocco E, Sacerdote P, Mantegazza P. Dissociation of tolerance and dependence to morphine: A possible role for cholecystokinin. *Brain Res* 1987; 410: 52-60.

4. Dourish CT, Hawley D, Iversen SD. Enhancement of morphine analgesia and prevention of morphine tolerance in the rat by the cholecystokinin antagonist L364,718. *Eur J Pharmacol* 1988; 147: 469-472.

5. Dourish CT, O'Neill MF, Coughlan J, Kitchener SJ, Hawley D, Iversen SD. The selective CCK-B receptor antagonist L365,260 enhances morphine analgesia and prevents morphine tolerance in the rat. *Eur J Pharmacol* 1990; 176: 35-44.

6. Idanpaan-Heikkila JJ, Guilbaud G, Kayser V. Prevention of tolerance to the antinociceptive effects of systemic morphine by a selective cholecystokinin-B receptor antagonist in a rat model of peripheral neuropathy. *J Pharmacol Exp Ther* 1997; 282 : 1366-1372.

7. Vinik HR, Kissin I. Rapid development of tolerance to analgesia during remifentanil infusion in humans. *Anesth Analg* 1998; 86: 1307 0-11.

8. Kissin I, Lee SS, Arthur GR, Bradley EL. Time course characteristics of acute tolerance development to continuously infused alfentanil in rats. *Anesth Analg* 1996; 83: 600-605.

9. Bilsky EJ, Inturrisi CE, Sadee W et al. Competitive and non-competitive NMDA antagonists block the development of antinociceptive tolerance to morphine, but not to selective mu or delta opioid agonists in mice. *Pain* 1995; 68: 229-237.

10. Kissin I, Bright CA, Bradley EL. Acute tolerance to continuously infused alfentanil: The role of cholecystokinin and N-methyl-D-aspartate-nitric oxide systems. *Anesth Analg* 2000; 91: 110-116.

11. Holladay KM, Lin CW. CCK agonist: A summary of structure-activity relationships with a focus on A-71378, a potent selective CCK-A agonist. *Drug Future* 1992; 17: 197-206.

12. Slaninova J, Knapp RJ, Wu J et al. Opioid receptor binding properties of analgesic analogues of cholecystokinin octapeptide. *Eur J Pharmacol* 1991; 200: 195-198.

13. Zarrindast M-R, Zabihi A, Rezayat M, Rakhshandeh H, Ghazi-Khansari M, Hosseini R. Effects of caerulein and CCK antagonists on tolerance induced to morphine antinociception in mice. *Pharmacol Biochem Behav* 1997; 58: 173-178.

14. Barbaz BS, Autry WL, Ambrose FG, Hall NR, Liebman JM. Antinociceptive profile of sulphated CCK-8. *Neuropharmacology* 1986; 25: 823-829.

15. Hill RG, Hughes J, Pittaway KM. Antinociceptive action of cholecystokinin octapeptide (CCK-8) and related peptides in rats and mice: Effects of naloxone and peptidase inhibitors. *Neuropharmacology* 1987; 26: 289-300.

16. Zarrindast M-R, Malekzadeh A, Rezayat M, Ghazi-Khansari M. Effects of cholecystokinin receptor agonist and antagonists on morphine dependence in mice. *Pharmacol Toxiciol* 1995; 77: 360-365.

17. Zetler G. Cholecystokinin octapeptide, caerulein and caerulein analogues: Effect on thermoregulation in the mouse. *Neuropharmacology* 1982; 21: 795-801.

18. Zarrindast M-R, Nifkar S, Rezayat M. Cholecystokinin receptor mechanism(s) and morphine tolerance in mice. *Pharmacol Toxicol* 1999; 84: 46-50.

19. Hoffmann O, Wiesenfeld-Hallin Z. The CCK-B receptor antagonist CI988 reverses tolerance to morphine in rats. *NeuroReport* 1994; 5: 2565-2568.

20. Ding XZ, Fan SG, Zhou JP et al. Reversal of tolerance but no potentiation of morphine-induced analgesia by antiserum against cholecystokinin octapeptide. *Neuropharmacology* 1986; 25: 1155-1160.

21. Rezvani A, Stokes BK, Rhoads DL et al. Proglumide exhibits delta opioid agonist properties. *Alc Drug Res* 1987; 7: 135-146.

22. Holaday JW, Hitzemann RJ, Curell J et al. Repeated electroconvulsive shock or chronic morphine treatment increases the number of 3H-D-Ala^7,D-Leu^5-enkephalin binding sites in rat brain membranes. *Life Sci* 1982; 31: 2359-2362.

23. Hughes J, Boden P, Costall B et al. Development of a class of selective cholecystokinin type B receptor antagonists having potent anxiolytic activity. *Proc Natl Acad Sci USA* 1990; 87: 6728-6732.

24. Tortorici V, Nogueira L, Salas R, Vanegas H. Involvement of local cholecystokinin in the tolerance induced by morphine microinjection into the periaqueductal gray of rats. *Pain* 2003; 102: 9-16.

25. Siuciak JA, Advokat C. Tolerance to morphine microinjections in the periaqueductal gray (PAG) induces tolerance to systemic, but not to intrathecal morphine. *Brain Res* 1987; 424: 311-319.

26. Tortorici V, Morgan MM, Vanegas H. Tolerance to repeated microinjections of morphine into the periaqueductal gray is associated with changes of the behaviour of off- and on- cells in the rostral ventromedial medulla. *Pain* 2000; 89: 237-244.

27. Vaughan CW, Ingram SL, Connor MA, Christie MJ. How opioids inhibit GABA-mediated neurotransmission. *Nature* 1997; 390: 611-616.

28. Fields HL, Basbaum AI. Central nervous system mechanisms of pain modulation. In PD Wall, R Melzack (Eds.), *Textbook of pain* (Fourth ed.) (pp. 309-329). London: Churchill Livingstone, 1999.

29. Fields HL, Heinricher MM, Mason P. Neurotransmitters in nociceptive modulatory circuits. *Annu Rev Neurosci* 1991; 14: 219-245.

30. Fields HL, Malick A, Burstein R. Dorsal horn projection targets of ON and OFF cells in the rostral ventromedial medulla. *J Neurophysiol* 1995; 74: 1742-1759.

31. Miller KK, Hoffer A, Svoboda KR, Lupica CR. Cholecystokinin increases GABA release by inhibiting a resting K^+ conductance in hippocampal interneurons. *J Neurosci* 1997; 17: 4994-5003.

32. Mitchell JM, Basbaum AI, Fields HL. A locus and mechanism of action for associative morphine tolerance. *Nature Neuroscience* 2000; 3: 47-53.

33. Pu S, Zhuang H, Lu Z, Wu X, Han J. Cholecystokinin gene expression in rat amygdaloid neurons: Normal distribution and effect of morphine tolerance. *Brain Res Mol Brain Res* 1994; 21: 183-189.

Chapter 12

1. Dourish CT, O'Neill MF, Schaffer LW, Siegl PK, Iversen SD. The cholecystokinin receptor antagonist devazepide enhances morphine-induced analgesia but not morphine-induced respiratory depression in the squirrel monkey. *J Pharmacol Exp Ther* 1990; 255: 1158-1165.

2. Hill DR, Shaw TM, Woodruff GN. Binding sites for ^{125}I-cholecystokinin in primate spinal cord are of the CCK-A subclass. *Neurosci Lett* 1988; 7: 133-139.

3. McCleane GJ. A phase 1 study of the cholecystokinin (CCK) B antagonist L365,260 in human subjects taking morphine for intractable non-cancer pain. *Neurosci Lett* 2002; 332: 210-212.

Chapter 13

1. Price DD, von der Gruen A, Miller J, Rafii A, Price C. Potentiation of systemic morphine analgesia in humans by proglumide, a cholecystokinin antagonist. *Anesth Analg* 1985; 64: 801-806.

2. Lavigne GJ, Hargreaves KM, Schmidt EA, Dionne RA. Proglumide potentiates morphine analgesia for acute postsurgical pain. *Clin Pharmacol Ther* 1989; 45: 666-673.

3. Watkins LR, Kinscheck IB, Mayer DJ. Potentiation of opiate analgesia and apparent reversal of morphine tolerance by proglumide. *Science* 1984; 224: 395-396.

4. Watkins LR, Kinscheck IB, Mayer DJ. Potentiation of morphine analgesia by the cholecystokinin antagonist proglumide. *Brain Res* 1985; 327: 169-180.

5. Lehmann KA, Schlusener M, Arabatsis P. Failure of proglumide, a cholecystokinin antagonist, to potentiate clinical morphine analgesia. *Anesth Analg* 1989; 68: 51-56.

6. Bernsetein ZP, Yucht S, Battista E, Lema M, Spaulding MB. Proglumide as a morphine adjunct in cancer pain management. *J Pain Sympt Manage* 1998; 15: 314-320.

7. McCleane GJ. The cholecystokinin antagonist proglumide enhances the analgesic effect of morphine in chronic benign nociceptive and neuropathic pain. *Pain Clinic* 1998; 11: 103-107.

8. McCleane GJ. The cholecystokinin antagonist proglumide enhances the analgesic efficacy of morphine in humans with chronic benign pain. *Anesth Analg* 1998; 87: 1117-1120.

9. McCleane GJ. The cholecystokinin antagonist proglumide enhances the analgesic effect of dihydrocodeine. *Clin J Pain* 2003; 19: 200-201.

10. McCleane GJ. The cholecystokinin antagonist proglumide has an analgesic effect when used alone in human neuropathic pain: A case report. *Pain Clinic* 2003; 15: 71-73.

11. Rezani A, Stokes B, Rhoads DL, Way EL. Proglumide exhibits delta opioid agonist properties. *Alc Drug Res* 1987; 7: 135-146.

12. Valverde O, Maldonado R, Fournie-Zaluski MC, Roques BP. Cholecystokinin B antagonists strongly potentiate antinociception mediated by endogenous enkephalins. *J Pharmacol Exp Ther* 1994; 270: 77-88.

13. Noble F, Derrien M, Roques BP. Modulation of opioid antinociception by CCK at the supra-spinal level: Evidence of regulatory mechanisms between CCK and enkephalin systems in the control of pain. *Br J Pharmacol* 1993; 109: 1064-1070.

14. Vanderah TW, Bernstein RN, Lai J, Porreca F. Production of naltrindole-sensitive antinociception by a cholecystokinin (CCK) antagonist and thiorphan: Evidence for tonic inhibition of enkephalin release by CCK. *Analgesia* 1995; 1: 813-816.

15. McCleane GJ. A randomised, double-blind, placebo controlled crossover study of the cholecystokinin 2 antagonist L365,260 as an adjunct to strong opioids in chronic human neuropathic pain. *Neurosci Lett* 2003; 338: 151-154.

16. Hill DR, Shaw TM, Graham W, Woodruff GN. Auto radiographic detection of cholecystokinin-A receptors in primate brain using ^{125}I-Bolton Hunter CCK8 and ^{3}H-MK-329. *J Neurosci* 1990; 10: 1070-1081.

17. Suh HW, Kim Y-H, Choi YS, Song DK. Involvement of different subtypes of cholecystokinin receptors in opioid antinociception in the mouse. *Peptides* 1995; 16: 1229-1234.

18. Yamamoto N, Nozaki-Taguchi N. The effects of intrathecally administered FK480, a cholecystokinin A receptor antagonist, and YM022, a cholecystokinin B receptor antagonist, on the formalin test in the rat. *Anesth Analg* 1996; 83: 107-113.

19. Simpson KH, Serpell M, McCubbins TD et al. A multi-dose study: Management of neuropathic pain in patients using a CCK antagonist devazepide (Devacade) as an adjunct to strong opioids. Abstract. World Congress on Pain, San Diego, 2002: 479. IASP Press, Seattle.

20. McCleane GJ. The cholecystokinin antagonist proglumide reduces analgesic tolerance to morphine in humans with chronic benign pain. *Pain Clinic* 1999; 11: 309-312.

21. Pahl IR, Koppert W, Enk C et al. Different lipid profiles as constituencies of liquid formula diets do not influence pain perception and the efficacy of opioids in a human model of acute pain and hyperalgesia. *Pain* 2003; 104: 519-527.

22. Zhu XG, Greeley Jr GH, Lewis BG, Lilja P, Thompson JC. Blood-CSF barrier to CCK and effect of centrally administered bombesin on release of brain CCK. *J Neurosci Res* 1986; 15: 393-403.

23. Makovec F, Bani M, Chiste R, Revel L, Rovati LC, Rovati LA. Differentiation of central and peripheral cholecystokinin receptors by new glutaramic acid

derivatives with cholecystokinin-antagonistic activity. *Arzneim-Forsch Drug Res* 1986; 36: 98-102.

Chapter 14

1. Liddle RA, Goldfine ID, Rosen MS, Taplitz RA, Williams JA. Cholecystokinin bioactivity in human plasma: Molecular forms, responses to feeding, and relationship to gallbladder contractions. *J Clin Invest* 1985; 75: 1144-1152.

2. Konturek JW, Konturek SJ, Kurek A, Bogdal J, Olesky J, Rovati L. CCK receptor antagonism by loxiglumide and gallbladder contractions in response to cholecystokinin, sham feeding and ordinary feeding in man. *Gut* 1989; 30: 1136-1142.

3. Liddle RA, Gertz BJ, Kanayama S et al. Effects of a novel cholecystokinin (CCK) receptor antagonist, MK-329, on gallbladder contraction and gastric emptying in humans. *J Clin Invest* 1989; 84: 1220-1225.

4. Cantor P, Mortensen E, Myhre J et al. The effect of the cholecystokinin receptor antagonist MK-329 on meal-stimulated pancreaticobiliary output in humans. *Gastroenterology* 1992; 102: 1242-1251.

5. Malesci A, Pezzilli R, D'Amato M, Rovati L. CCK-1 receptor blockade for treatment of biliary colic: A pilot study. *Aliment Pharmacol Ther* 2003; 18: 333-337.

6. Funakoshi A, Nakano I, Shinozaki H et al. Low plasma cholecystokinin response after ingestion of a test meal in patients with chronic pancreatitis. *Am J Gastroenterol* 1985; 80: 937-940.

7. Eddes EH, Masclee AA, Gielkens HA et al. Cholecystokinin secretion in patients with chronic pancreatitis and after different types of pancreatic surgery. *Pancreas* 1999; 19: 119-125.

8. Nakamura T, Tando Y, Yamada N et al. Meal-related changes in plasma CCK bioactivity in patients with chronic pancreatitis. *Acta Gastro Enterol Belg* 1998; 61: 400-406.

9. Hirano H, Shimosegawa T, Meguro T et al. Effects of ethanol on meal-stimulated secretion of pancreatic polypeptide and cholecystokinin: Comparison of healthy volunteers, heavy drinkers, and patients with chronic pancreatitis. *J Gastroenterol* 1996; 31: 86-93.

10. Schafmayer A, Becker HD, Werner M, Folsch UR, Creutzfeldt W. Plasma cholecystokinin levels in patients with chronic pancreatitis. *Digestion* 1985; 32: 136-139.

11. Garces MC, Gomez-Cerezo J, Codoceo R, Grande C, Barbado J, Vazquez J-J. Postprandial cholecystokinin response in patients with chronic pancreatitis in treatment with oral substitutive pancreatic enzymes. *Digest Dis Sci* 1998; 43: 562-566.

12. Ederle A, Vantini I, Harvey RF et al. Fasting serum cholecystokinin immunoreactivity in chronic relapsing pancreatitis. *La Ricera Clin Lab* 1978; 8: 199-206.

13. Garces MC, Gomez-Cerezo J, Alba D et al. Relationship of basal and postprandial intraduodenal bile acid concentrations and plasma cholecystokinin levels with abdominal pain in patients with chronic pancreatitis. *Pancreas* 1998; 17: 397-401.

14. Gomez-Cerezo J, Codoceo R, Calle PF, Molina F, Tenias JM, Vazquez. Basal and postprandial cholecystokinin values in chronic pancreatitis with and without abdominal pain. *Digestion* 1991; 48: 134-140.

15. McCleane GJ. The cholecystokinin antagonist proglumide has an analgesic effect in chronic pancreatitis. *Pancreas* 2000; 21: 324-325.

16. Watanabe O, Baccino FM, Steer ML, Meldolisi J. Supramaximal caerulein stimulation and ultrastructure of rat pancreatic acinar cells: Early morphological changes during development of experimental pancreatitis. *Am J Physiol* 1984; 246: G457-467.

17. Saluja A, Saito I, Saluja M et al. In vivo rat acinar cell function during submaximal stimulation with caerulein. *Am J Physiol* 1985; 249: G702-710.

18. Evander A, Ihse I, Lundquist I. Influence of gastrointestinal hormones on the course of acute experimental pancreatitis. *Hepato Gastroenterol* 1982; 29: 161-166.

19. Evander A, Ihse I. Influence of hormonal stimulation by caerulein on acute experimental pancreatitis in rats. *Eur Surg Res* 1981; 13: 257-268.

20. Niederau C, Liddle RA, Ferrel LD, Grendell JH. Beneficial effects of cholecystokinin receptor blockage and inhibition of proteolytic enzyme activity in experimental acute hemorrhagic pancreatitis in mice: Evidence for cholecystokinin as a major factor in the development of acute pancreatitis. *J Clin Invest* 1986; 78: 1056-1063.

21. Niederau C, Ferrel LD, Grendell JH. Caerulein-induced acute necrotizing pancreatitis in mice: Protective effect of proglumide, benzotript and secretin. *Gastroenterol* 1985; 88: 1192-1204.

22. Makovec F, Bani M, Cereda R et al. Protective effect of CR1409 (cholecystokinin antagonist) on experimental pancreatitis in rats and mice. *Peptide* 1986; 7: 1159-1164.

23. Tani S, Okabayashi Y, Nakamura T, Fujii M, Otsuki M. Effect of a new cholecystokinin receptor antagonist loxiglumide on acute pancreatitis in two animal experimental models. *Pancreas* 1990; 5: 284-290.

24. Leonhardt U, Seidensticher F, Fussek M, Stockman F, Creutzfeld W. Influence of the CCK-antagonist loxiglumide on bile-induced experimental pancreatitis. *Int J Pancreatol* 1991; 10: 73-80.

25. Satake K, Kimura K, Saito T. Therapeutic effects of loxiglumide on experimental acute pancreatitis using various models. *Digestion* 1999; 60: S64-68.

26. Netto CF, Guimaraes FS. Anxiogenic effect of cholecystokinin in the dorsal periaqueductal gray. *Neuropsychopharmacol* 2004; 29: 101-107.

27. De Montigny C. Cholecystokinin tetrapeptide induces panic like attacks in healthy volunteers: Preliminary findings. *Arch Gen Psychiatry* 1989; 46: 511-517.

28. Abelson JL, Neese R. Cholecystokinin-4 and panic. *Arch Gen Psychiatry* 1990; 47: 395P.

29. Bradwejn J, Koszycki D, Meterissian G. Cholecystokinin-tetrapeptide induces panic attacks in patients with panic disorder. *Can J Psychiatry* 1990; 35: 83-85.

30. Hendrie CA, Neill JC, Shepherd JK, Dourish CT. The effects of CCK A and CCK B antagonists on activity in the black/white exploration model of anxiety in mice. *Physiol Behav* 1993; 54: 689-693.

31. Hughes J, Boden P, Costall B et al. Development of a class of selective cholecystokinin type B receptor antagonists having potent anxiolytic activity. *Proc Natl Acad Sci USA* 1990; 87: 6728-6732.

32. Motta V, Brandao ML. Aversive and anti-aversive effects of morphine in the dorsal periaqueductal gray of rats submitted to elevated plus-maze test. *Pharmacol Biochem Behav* 1993; 44: 119-125.

33. Koks S, Soosaar A, Voikar V et al. Opioid antagonist naloxone potentiates anxiogenic-like action of cholecystokinin agonists in elevated plus-maze. *Neuropeptides* 1998; 32: 235-240.

34. Koks S, Soosaar A, Voikar V, Bourin M, Vasar E. BOC-CCK-4, CCK B receptor agonist, antagonizes anxiolytic-like action of morphine in elevated plus-maze. *Neuropeptides* 1999; 33: 63-69.

35. Bickerdike MJ, Marsden CA, Dourish CT, Fletcher A. The influence of 5-hydroxytryptamine re-uptake blockade on CCK receptor antagonist effect in the rat elevated zero-maze. *Eur J Pharmacol* 1994; 271: 403-411.

36. Raiteri M, Paudice P, Vallebuona F. Inhibition by 5HT$_3$ receptor antagonists of release of cholecystokinin-like immunoreactivity from the frontal cortex of freely moving rats. *Naunyn Schmied Arch Pharmacol* 1993; 347: 111.

37. Rex A, Fink H, Marsden CA. The effect of CCK-4 and L365,260 on cortical extracellular 5-HT release on exposure on the elevated plus maze. In E Hamon, H Ollat and MH Theibot (Eds.), *Anxiety: Neurobiology, clinic and therapeutic perspectives* (pp. 207, 232). Colloque, France: INSERM / John Libbey Eurotext.

38. Vasar E, Peuranen E, Oopik T, Harro J, Mannisto PT. Ondansetron, an antagonist of 5-HT$_3$ receptors, antagonises the anti-exploratory effect of caerulein, an agonist of CCK receptors, in the elevated plus-maze test. *Psychopharmacology* 1993; 110: 213.

39. Lu L, Huang M, Liu Z, Ma L. Cholecystokinin-B receptor antagonists attenuate morphine dependence and withdrawal in rats. *NeuroReport* 2000; 11: 829-832.

40. Lu L, Huang M, Ma L, Li J. Different role of cholecystokinin (CCK)-A and CCK-B receptors in relapse to morphine dependence in rats. *Behav Brain Res* 2001; 105-110.

41. Valverde O, Roques BP. Cholecystokinin modulates the aversive component of morphine withdrawal syndrome in rats. *Neurosci Lett* 1998; 244: 37-40.

42. Rasmussen K, Helton DR, Berger JE, Scearce E. The CCK-B antagonist LY288513 blocks effects of diazepam withdrawal on auditory startle. *NeuroReport* 1993; 5: 154-156.

43. Harro J, Lang A, Vasar E. Long-term diazepam treatment produces changes in cholecystokinin receptor binding in the brain. *Eur J Pharmacol* 1990; 180: 77-83.

44. Rattray M, Singhvi S, Wu P-Y et al. Benzodiazepines increase preprocholecystokinin messenger RNA levels in rat brain. *Eur J Pharmacol Mol Pharm* 1993; 245: 193-196.

45. Singh L, Lewis AS, Filed MJ, Hughes J, Woodruff GN. Evidence for an involvement of the brain cholecystokinin B receptor in anxiety. *Proc Natl Acad Sci USA* 1991; 88: 1130-1133.

46. Hughes J, Boden P, Costall B et al. Development of a class of selective cholecystokinin type B receptor antagonists having potent anxiolytic activity. *Proc Natl Acad Sci USA* 1990; 87: 6728-6732.

47. Singh L, Field MJ, Vass CA, Hughes J, Woodruff GN. The antagonism of benzodiazepine withdrawal effects by the selective cholecystokinin B receptor antagonist CI-988. *Br J Pharmacol* 1992; 105: 8-10.

48. Panerai AE, Rovati LC, Bianchi M, Bareggi SR, Mantegazza P. Effect of a cholecystokinin antagonist on some effects of diazepam. *Neuropharmacol* 1987; 26: 1285-1287.

49. Wilson J, Woodruff GN, Little HJ. Concurrent chronic administration of a CCK B antagonist can decrease tolerance to the ataxic effects of ethanol. *Addiction Biol* 1999; 4: 35-45.

50. Wilson J, Watson WP, Little HJ. CCK B antagonists protect against anxiety-related behaviour produced by ethanol withdrawal, measured using the elevated plus maze. *Psychopharmacology* 1987; 137: 120-131.

51. Wilson J, Little HJ. CCK B antagonists protect against some aspects of the ethanol withdrawal syndrome. *Pharmacol Biochem Behav* 1998; 59: 967-973.

Index